PANIC = THE STORY OF AIDS

PANIC

THE STORY OF

AIDS

Robin McKie

with a Foreword by

Anthony Pinching

Clinical Immunologist
St Mary's Hospital Medical School

THORSONS PUBLISHING GROUP
Wellingborough • New York

First published 1986

British Library Cataloguing in Publication Data

McKie, Robin
  Panic : the story of AIDS.
  1. AIDS (Disease)
  I. Title
  616.9'792   RC607.A26

ISBN 0-7225-1340-2

Printed and bound in Great Britain

Contents

Foreword

The Acquired Immune Deficiency Syndrome (AIDS) and its causative virus have probably created more challenges to medicine, science and society than any other single disease. Many of these have been real but, others, sadly, have been spurious problems that have arisen only because of misinformation, misunderstanding and prejudice. The need for accurate and responsible reporting of medical matters has never been greater. This is of course primarily the job of journalists, subeditors and editors, but doctors and scientists must provide them with relevant information in a comprehensible, balanced and accurate form, not confusing facts with speculations. Yet AIDS has fallen victim to the same process that has bedevilled the public discussion of so many other medical matters, in which facts are distorted, overdramatized and oversimplified for the sake of making good entertainment. Discerning reporters have realized that the true story of AIDS has all the necessary ingredients to capture and retain the interest of the ordinary person. By pursuing the story accurately they can also ensure public education in this vital area of public health.

Of course the writing of any contemporary history must be subjective so there can certainly be no definitive way of telling this extraordinary and terrible story. The validity of any report from the 'front' ultimately rests on the ability of the writer not only to get so close to the action that he can smell the powder, but also to convey the feel of that action to his armchair reader. In this book, Robin McKie has managed to distil the most important and exciting aspects of this remarkable chapter in the story of human disease. He has done so in a form that is readable and informative without doing violence to truth. In doing it he has also allowed the flavour of the real problems — medical, scientific and social — to come across without the superfluous embellishment that others have deemed necessary.

When a new disease appears it is always disturbing to the public to think that we do not know very much about it. Certainly in the earliest days of this decade, there was justifiable concern about what was not known about AIDS. When it was realized that AIDS was the result of an unidentified infectious agent, even more alarm was generated, although by then we knew a lot about the way in which this unseen enemy was behaving. Now, after some five years of intensive study, we know more about AIDS and its causative virus than we know about many diseases that have been around for centuries. It is vital to convey this rapid increase in knowledge to the public, not only to allay unnecessary anxiety, but also to allow them to recognize the very real medical and social issues that arise from it. There is now no need to fear the unknown, even though much research still needs to be done, notably in prevention and treatment.

In the realm of science, AIDS demanded a swift and effective response to identify its causative agent and to determine how it causes disease. The response has indeed been quick, largely because it was possible to base the investigation on established methods of disease surveillance and on basic scientific techniques in virology, immunology and molecular biology. In some ways we were fortunate that the infection emerged when it did, because even ten years before the problems would have been immense. Much of the advantage resulted from substantial investment over recent years in basic scientific research; this investment was made recognizing that such basic information would ultimately be of practical value, even if we did not necessarily know how it would be applied. This point has important implications for the planning of future research, which we cannot afford to base solely on the problems that currently confront us.

Furthermore, AIDS has also shown us that some of our pre-existing scientific ideas were too narrowly conceived and formulated. The progress we have made in the investigation of AIDS has been achieved by cutting through a miasma of jargon and loose thinking. As is usual in any science, the fundamental truths are simple and can be expressed simply. Success has depended upon our ability to discern the simple but vital messages that our patients are revealing to us. For the fact is that all the basic scientific discoveries about AIDS, which have shed light both on this disease and many others, have resulted from listening to what the patients are telling us.

Medicine too has been challenged to refine its concepts, not only in recognizing new patterns of disease but also in treating our patients from the widest possible perspective. For AIDS has reminded us of the tremendous social and personal impact of disease, something that can only be handled through a very full appreciation of its significance in human terms. The term 'holistic medicine' has been hijacked by the proponents of alternative medicine as if it were fundamentally different from the objectives of conventional medical practice. Conventional medicine is certainly the poorer if it is anything less than holistic in outlook. AIDS has forcibly removed the blinkers from our view of our own medical practices; even if the experience may have been momentarily blinding, it can only be for the better in the treatment of all our patients. If we cannot appreciate the whole of a medical problem from the patient's perspective we cannot expect to provide effective treatment and support.

The need for a team approach to such a complex medical problem is self-evident. AIDS has underlined the need to involve all elements in the team as equals, each contributing his or her own special skills and qualities. The perception of AIDS as an infectious disease that could possibly pose an occupational threat to staff has reinforced the need for individual involvement in the vocation. This applies to levels of staff education, to basic principles of care in looking after sick people and to the special committment that underlies being a member of a caring profession. In these respects, AIDS has renewed lines of communication between different parts of the health care profession, so that doctors, nurses, ancillary staff and laboratory workers all recognize and understand their vital role in the care of patients. If this implies criticism of the way in which medicine has sometimes previously been practised, so be it. We are the better for it. While we can still respond to the challenges presented by ill people, while we can still learn how to do better, then there is hope for us all, be we consumers or providers of health care. Patients again are showing us the way.

Society too has been challenged by AIDS. Recent years have seen tremendous changes in the structure of society and in the behaviour and attitudes of those individuals who constitute it. AIDS and the perceptions that have surrounded it, both real and imagined, have really lifted the lid off society; they have enabled us to examine it and, through it, ourselves. The fear and the prejudice that have surrounded the problem of AIDS have been surprising and often horrifying. They have certainly raised the question as to whether we are as caring and tolerant as we may previously have imagined. We have learnt that under the thin veneer of permissiveness and broad-mindedness, there is a disturbingly solid mass of intolerance and prejudice. Even as individuals, we have sometimes found that the problems which confront us in AIDS have forced us to reassess our perceptions of ourselves; not everything we have discovered has been nice.

But if some of these comments, and indeed parts of this book, seem to cast a gloomy light over our society, we must not forget that there has been a very positive side. Scientists have shown a remarkable openness and readiness to co-operate in the fight against this tragic new disease, in a way that has generally been exemplary. The exceptions that you may read about are notable mainly because they are uncharacteristic. A personal commitment to the solution of the scientific problems has been a major factor in the speed of scientific discovery. Many health care professionals at all levels have responded to the challenge with tremendous skill, selfless personal effort and extraordinary compassion. Through their example we can avoid some previous errors. Finally many people in every section of society have shown that they are indeed compassionate and caring and that they are far too sensible to be misled by the scare stories. Their response has been a breath of fresh air.

Ultimately it is of course the patients and their loved ones who are the real and only true heroes of this story. You will find them populating Robin McKie's text with the natural sincerity and vulnerability of ordinary and yet extraordinary people. They need the best of us; if we deny it, then we too are the losers.

Anthony J. Pinching
BM BCh MA DPhil MRCP
Clinical Immunologist
St Mary's Hospital Medical School
LONDON

February 1986

1

Black Ghosts

In 1983, Dr Wilson Carswell, a Kampala-based physician noticed the first cases of a strange and deadly new illness among Ugandan citizens. Most victims were young adults, many came from rural areas, and all were suffering from drastic losses in weight — usually of around 3 to 4 stone (18 to 25 kg). In addition, most were covered with sores and skin infections. 'They looked like black ghosts, they were so desperately thin', recalls Dr Carswell. 'They would walk into surgeries looking like shadows, except for their lips which were bright white from the intense fungal infections in their mouths'. Chances of survival for these bizarrely disfigured young 'black ghosts' were dismal. The disease was remorseless and invariably fatal, causing its victims to waste to death.

The illness was mysterious and new to Dr Carswell, a Paisley-born British doctor who had worked in Uganda for fifteen years. He and his colleagues were baffled both by the sudden appearance of the disease and by its unusual virulence. Their attempts to find its cause were hampered, however, by the bitter civil war which then gripped Uganda. The resulting chaos prevented serious investigations of the epidemic. For their part, local Ugandans simply labelled the illness 'slim disease' and blamed it on witchcraft. But in 1985, a crucial breakthrough was made by an international team of scientists, working with help from Dr Carswell and his colleagues. Studying blood samples from victims, they found that nearly all had been infected with a virus known as HTLV3/LAV.

It was a startling discovery, for HTLV3/LAV is better known for its infamous Western associations — as the cause of AIDS, the immune disease which destroys victims' powers to fight various cancers and pneumonias. AIDS (now designated the number one health priority in the US) had already been discovered in Africa. But its link with slim disease, with which it has a great many common features, revealed a disturbing new dimension to the illness. In the US and Europe, AIDS (an acronym for Acquired Immune Deficiency Syndrome) primarily affects high risk groups: male homosexuals, drug takers who share needles, and haemophiliacs given infected blood products. The vast majority are men, and in most cases contaminated blood and genital secretions were thought to be the main transmission routes.

In Africa, men and women are affected by AIDS in almost equal numbers. Tribal scarring, the use of dirty needles by witchdoctors, and biting insects were variously put forward to account for the assumed exchange of blood and to explain the very different pattern of cases being found in Africa. But these notions were dealt a severe blow when it was found that few victims had been given recent injections or had tribal scars, while the high predominance of young, sexually active adults among cases ruled out insect bites (which would have affected people of all ages).

In fact, the main risk factor appeared simply to be promiscuous behaviour. The inference was clear. AIDS was really a standard sexually transmitted disease — though of a particularly deadly variety. 'Having ruled out everything else, we concluded that AIDS is spread through heterosexual activity', says one of the investigators, Dr Angus Dalgleish, of London's Institute of Cancer Research.

This view was endorsed by the distinguished French scientist, Dr Nathan Clumeck, of the St Pierre Hospital, University of Brussels, and the organizer of the first International Symposium on African AIDS, held in November 1985. 'Some people still believe that insects are involved. Some say that unsterilized needles play a role. I think that it is much simpler than that. In Africa, as in America and Europe, the virus is mostly transmitted by sexual contact'.

Such interpretations were shared by growing numbers of other scientists in Europe and the US. They were becoming alarmed by the number of cases of AIDS appearing in the general population. Victims included wives of AIDS patients, prostitutes, and sometimes their clients. The disease was clearly moving out of groups who were previously thought to be the only ones at risk. It was, and is, a highly disturbing development. AIDS spread through central Africa in a few years, affecting both men and women in the process. Now Europe and the United States face a similar threat. Most senior scientists are extremely worried, including Dr Robert Gallo, co-discoverer of HTLV3/LAV and one of America's leading AIDS experts. 'AIDS is emerging as the most lethal pandemic of the second half of the twentieth century', he wrote in the distinguished science journal *Nature* in late 1985. (A pandemic is defined as an epidemic so widely spread that vast numbers of people in different countries are affected.)

It is a chilling development. In five years, a previously unknown disease has acquired a scientific reputation which rivals those of cholera, the plague, polio, syphilis, and influenza — all killers of millions of people in the past. Doctors have been caught completely off guard. Even more so, the attitudes of our so-called sophisticated Western society have been found to be badly wanting. Fuelled by hysterical newspaper reporting, large sections of the population have embarked on witch-hunts of suspected AIDS virus carriers, a course of action with depressing historical parallels. Jews were blamed for the Black Death; Irish immigrants for the last century's New York yellow fever outbreak; and the Hungarian aristocracy for deliberately spreading cholera in the 1830s.

Now homosexuals (and to a lesser extent drug takers and haemophiliacs) are at the receiving end of similar bigotry generated by ignorance. Gays are being spat at and punched in the street; others are being sacked as potential AIDS risks; while those found to be carrying the virus may be refused life insurance, mortgages and accommodation.

'These reactions are deep rooted' says Jonathan Grimshaw, founder of Body Positive, a British support group for AIDS virus carriers. 'AIDS is associated with death, lingering illness and sexuality — all themes that people wish to keep furthest from their thoughts. They bitterly resent being made aware of them'.

Such prejudice is only made worse by newspapers which continually refer to AIDS as a 'gay plague'. This is quite incorrect: AIDS is neither 'gay' nor is it a 'plague'. Many heterosexual men and women are now infected, while touching, sharing a cup, or sitting close to a victim, carry no risk (though they might with the plague). AIDS can only be transmitted through intimate activities involving the exchange of blood, semen, or genital secretions. Yet people persistently ignore such assurances and continue to persecute gays. Fear and prejudice have become all too familiar features of the experiences of gays, and of the researchers and counsellors who are working to help victims.

'I think the emergence of AIDS has finally killed off any idea that we live in a caring, liberal or understanding society', says one of Britain's top AIDS experts, Dr Tony Pinching, an immunologist at St Mary's Hospital, London and author of the foreword to this book. 'We are just as prejudiced as we have always been. There is no shortage of people who refuse to take a rational view of fellow men and women who are suffering from a terrible ailment'.

This prejudice has frightening implications because AIDS has probably become a fixed feature of modern life. Preventing its further spread, and coping with thousands of new victims, will require a far calmer and more rational approach than exists today. At present, there may be almost two million US citizens who carry the AIDS virus in their blood and between ten and fifty thousand in Britain. Other Western nations are affected in similar proportions. At least 10 per cent of these carriers will contract the full, usually fatal, AIDS. Many of the rest may well suffer ill-health for the rest of their lives (which may be shortened in the process) although an unknown proportion may remain well. Dealing with such widespread tragedy will strain even the richest nation's health resources.

Worse still, this alarming scenario does not take into account the disease's continuing spread, although such an increase seems inevitable. Those who carry the AIDS virus are considered by scientists to be infected, and infectious, for the rest of their lives. The virus appears to live indefinitely in the blood cells of those infected. This means that a permanent pool of AIDS carriers has already been created throughout much of the world, one that can infect new victims at any time.

And treating these infected carriers may prove to be remarkably difficult. Scientists have recently found that the AIDS virus may also infect the brain and central nervous system. This means that the virus can get inside the 'blood–brain barrier', the mechanism which separates the circulating blood from the tissues of our brains. Solid particles and large molecules cannot pass through this barrier — which means that effective anti-AIDS drugs will have to be designed to get through the blood–brain barrier otherwise some viruses may be able to lurk within it, inside carriers' brains, ready to reinfect them at any time.

Indeed, the problem of brain damage caused by the AIDS virus is a new and potential devastating one. Scientists have discovered that the virus can not only cripple victims' immune systems but can also affect speech, sight, muscle co-ordination and awareness. One group of doctors, writing in *Nature* in January 1986, warned that in this century, in the US alone between a hundred thousand and one million people may suffer severe brain damage caused by the AIDS virus. An editorial in the journal urged caution, though it added that it believed the report was worth taking seriously. 'There is a possibility that HTLV3/LAV will lodge in infected people's brains, serving both as a cause of direct neurological damage and as a reservoir for the infection of others'. The consequences may be horrifying. As yet, there is no cure nor vaccine for AIDS. Only preventive measures can control its spread, one of the most urgent being to counsel against promiscuous behaviour. Yet such a reduction in sexual partnering will be extraordinarily difficult to achieve, given the important role that sex plays in most people's lives. As the American magazine *Newsweek* asked in September 1985: 'How can we realistically expect two million Americans to give up sex?'

For an answer, it is worth examining the efforts made by homosexuals, at present still the main group at risk of getting AIDS. In the United States, campaigns for 'safer sex' (intimate activities that do not involve the exchange of infected blood or semen) have had reasonable success, say doctors. Rates of venereal disease among homosexuals, an indicator of their promiscuity, have been greatly reduced. It is an encouraging sign, both for heterosexuals and for homosexuals in countries as yet unaffected by AIDS epidemics. But hope should be balanced with knowledge about the behaviour of the AIDS virus, which can remain in a victim's blood for years before producing its first symptoms. Many gays in San Francisco and New York were infectious without knowing it and only reduced their promiscuity when it was too late. They had already spread the virus unwittingly to other homosexuals. Now, three-quarters of San Francisco's gays are infected with the virus. In a few years, more than 10,000 of the city's young men will die as a result. In many US cities, AIDS is now the main cause of death among young adult males.

Clearly, early measures are needed to contain AIDS. In Europe, and in parts of the US outside large cities, it is not too late, even for gays. However, there is still no real sense of urgency, nor awareness of the real risks, nor knowledge about AIDS among a public that is still fixated with the notion that it is a 'plague' that might be picked up from a toilet seat. This has led some scientists and doctors to begin pressing for the introduction of compulsory measures, particularly ones to widen the use of newly developed tests which show if a person has been infected with the AIDS virus.

Their main target is the gay population. By preventing AIDS from spreading from homosexuals to bridging groups, such as bisexuals and prostitutes (who often use drugs), the main population may be protected, they argue. One suggested measure is to set up a 'green card' system for gays. The card would show that a person was free of the virus and safe as a potential sexual partner. Another measure would involve rigorously tracking all past partners of people found to be virus carriers. Then they too could be tested for the virus. Most homosexuals are appalled by such ideas. 'Gays have only recently become accepted as normal citizens', argues Tony Whitehead, chairman of the Terrence Higgins Trust, Britain's main support group for AIDS patients. 'Now people want to introduce cards that gays would need to carry before they were allowed to have sex. It would be like giving them pink triangles like the ones homosexuals had to wear in Hitler's concentration camps.'

Others warn that if virus-carrying gays were obliged to reveal details of all their past partners, many would simply refuse to take the test in the first place. AIDS carriers would be driven underground and the disease would become even harder to detect and control. Ensuring that effective preventive measures are taken while civil liberties (particularly for already hard-pressed minorities) are protected, will be extremely difficult. Nevertheless, an attempt is urgently needed before AIDS spreads much further.

Many European countries at last are taking action by introducing health education campaigns, widespread voluntary testing and other measures. Yet they have known about AIDS for five years and have watched the disease reach epidemic proportions in Africa and the US while doing nothing. A paralysis, induced by complacency and by a fear of causing panic and prejudice, has allowed those five years to be wasted. Now the situation has reached a critical state.

It is against this background of urgency that the story of AIDS should be read.

2

First Victims

The story of AIDS has all the ingredients of a racy detective novel. A few initially innocuous events that combine to baffle detectives; a lonely group of doomed victims; and a relentless, silent killer that mercilessly brings down its prey. And like all good detective stories, the villain is unmasked in a suitably dramatic denouement. Only the story of AIDS has an extra, unpleasant twist. The killer has continued its deadly business without pause.

This is the story of how the disease was tracked down and of how it affected its first victims. The tale begins in April 1981 at the US Centers for Disease Control (CDC), the Atlanta headquarters of the federal agency that is responsible for monitoring the health of the population of America. There, two scientists made a curious observation. It meant little at the time, though it did suggest that a strange new illness was afoot in America. The scientists could not know that the illness's potential was 'worse than anything mankind has seen before', as one of their senior colleagues, Dr Ward Cates stated four years later.

The discovery of the two researchers, Michael Gottlieb of the University of California in Los Angeles and Wayne Shandera of the CDC, was a simple one. They noticed a common thread to a handful of reports that had been sent to the CDC by doctors in New York and Los Angeles over the preceding months. Their first study, for the CDC's *Morbidity and Mortality Weekly Report,* was based on only five cases. Nevertheless, they provided enough information to cause interest. They showed that some, normally healthy, young gay men were suffering a breakdown of central parts of their immune system, the body's natural defences for countering infections. This was revealed through their contraction of diseases such as pneumonia, caused by a parasite called pneumocystis carinii (PCP). Shortly after this, another colleague, Harold Jaffe, found similar cases among San Francisco gays, though many were also suffering from another rare disease, a cancer, Kaposi's sarcoma, which attacks skin and internal organs.

These were a puzzling combination of ailments. Usually Kaposi's sarcoma only affects older men of Jewish and Mediterranean origins, while PCP is a normally rare lung infection caused by parasites. PCP caused a fatal outbreak of pneumonia among underfed, sickly refugee children at the end of the Second World War but rarely affects healthy adults. Immune breakdowns mainly occur in children afflicted by very uncommon genetic disorders or in patients specially treated by drugs so their bodies will not reject transplanted organs, such as kidneys or hearts.

The immune system is a highly sophisticated defence system that can mount a variety of different counter-attacks against organisms that invade the body. The discovery of this system's destruction in so many previously healthy young men was enough to cause concern at the CDC and to trigger a search for more information. Jaffe and his colleagues sought more cases — and quickly found them. In Atlanta, Los Angeles and Miami, cities with high populations of homosexuals, doctors were beginning to report more and more cases of gays who were afflicted by the same puzzling immune breakdowns. Victims were left powerless to fight a variety of different illnesses. Many died within a few months. (These effects gave rise to the name Acquired Immune Deficiency Syndrome: *acquired* means victims do not inherit the condition but catch it; *immune deficiency* implies they cannot fight diseases properly; and *syndrome* covers the rag bag of different infections typical of this condition.)

By summer 1981, the first alarm was being felt by CDC staff. Jaffe began searching through cancer patients' records and through request notices for the drug pentamidine, which is used to treat the pneumonia PCP. As he suspected, the immune disease was not new. There had been unrecognized cases occurring as far back as 1978. The CDC had only stumbled across AIDS when there were enough cases to be noticed by the center's staff. An epidemic was clearly beginning. But why were homosexuals the only ones to be affected by this new killer? Doctors suggested various causes: infection by a new virus or bacterium; the involvement of a bad batch of amyl nitrites, or 'poppers', which gays use as sexual stimulants; or straightforward collapses of homosexuals' immune systems after years of suffering infections provoked by promiscuous behaviour. (Doctors called this overloading.)

An immediate investigation was launched. Teams of scientists began to interview homosexuals, handing out questionnaires in the streets of gay districts. Others went to bath-houses, used by gays as centres for sexual pick-ups, while a few bought samples of poppers for testing. It was certainly an exotic change from normal laboratory work. 'Sometimes I felt I was in a Fellini movie — walking into Spanish Harlem, buying drugs, going to bath-houses', said one of the scientists in an interview in the journal *Science 83*. The task-force quickly realized that poppers could not be involved. They were used by far too many homosexuals to be the cause of AIDS. However, the team did find important clues. AIDS victims were found to have had many more sexual partners than uninfected homosexuals. The latter averaged twenty-five partners a year, AIDS victims about sixty, some reaching astonishing levels of several hundred. The evidence supported both the virus and the overload theories.

Then in autumn 1981, the first cases involving heterosexual men and women were reported. At Montefiore Hospital, in the sleazy Bronx district of New York, a doctor there, Gerald Friedland, discovered several intravenous drug users who had contracted PCP and other opportunistic infections. It was a strong indication that a mystery micro-organism was causing AIDS.

Drug addicts frequently share needles, passing syringes of heroin, or heroin substitutes, from addict to addict in large groups called 'shooting galleries'. Each time a needle is inserted into a vein blood is drawn back into the syringe. Some blood is then passed on to the next addict. If there is contamination, it is also passed on. In this way, many illnesses, such as hepatitis, are spread among drug users. Surely, a virus, or possibly a bacterium, was spreading AIDS in a similar way, argued doctors. The evidence was suggestive but not conclusive. Drug addicts suffer very poor health and other doctors maintained they could also be afflicted by immune overloads in the same way as gays. Clearer proof still was needed.

It came in January 1982. A haemophiliac from Miami was found to be suffering from PCP. He later died. Shortly after this, two other haemophiliacs died of similar AIDS-related illnesses. It was a crucial, and frightening, development. Haemophiliacs lack a blood-clotting substance called factor VIII. To prevent them from bleeding to death, they are given injections of factor VIII which is derived from the blood of donors. Often a single injection is derived from the blood of several thousand donors. In the case of the three haemophiliacs with AIDS, a donor must have infected their factor VIII. Most doctors now agreed that a mystery bug, probably a virus, was the only plausible candidate. But what really alarmed them, was the realization that the bug had begun to infect the blood banks of America.

The final confirmation that a micro-organism was involved in the spread of AIDS was provided by neat detective work by the CDC investigators. Hearing tales that many AIDS victims from Los Angeles had had sexual intercourse with each other before contracting the disease, Jaffe and his colleagues began a series of detailed interviews, compiling accounts of victims' behaviour and lovers. One day in early 1982, they made a remarkable breakthrough.

David Auerbach, a CDC officer, and Bill Darrow, one of the center's sociologists, interviewed an AIDS victim from nearby Orange County. He told them that he had had intercourse with a New York man with Kaposi's sarcoma. That afternoon the two researchers interviewed a second AIDS victim. Among his past lovers was the same New York sarcoma case named by the Orange County homosexual. It was an intriguing connection, but a more startling revelation was to follow. That evening, the two men continued their work. They interviewed a third AIDS patient. To their amazement, he too named the same New York gay as a past lover.

'These three men had never met, never had sex, yet they named the same guy in New York', recalls Darrow. 'I actually dropped my pen, Auerbach's mouth was just hanging open and he practically fell off his chair'. The cause of AIDS was clearly a transmissible micro-organism, through intimate contact or from sharing dirty needles — and perhaps through other routes. The CDC had established an important clue about the disease's behaviour.

By now AIDS was spreading in a very worrying manner. At the beginning of 1982, only nine months after the CDC had first heard about the disease, there were 216 cases on their records. Of these 88 were already dead. In addition, doctors were discovering cases of another related condition, known as lymphadenopathy. Sufferers were affected by swollen lymph glands, tiredness, night chills and sweats, fevers and sudden weight loss. Doctors suspected it was an early stage of AIDS. In the months that followed, other groups began to fall prey to AIDS. Firstly, large numbers of Haitians were diagnosed. (Haiti is a popular holiday resort with American gays.) Then came women who were sexual partners of victims. A little later doctors found that some of the women's babies had also contracted AIDS. By the end of 1982, twenty-six US children had been discovered to be suffering from the disease. Of these, ten were already dead.

The statistics were producing a numbing effect. But for

those affected, the tragedy was all too real and horrifying. All had to face the prospect of lingering illness and death. In addition, some had to suffer rejection and recrimination from friends, families and lovers. US magazines and newspapers were soon filled with their stories.

Andrew fared better than some. His family knew about his homosexuality and was perhaps better prepared than others when he became sick. In the summer of 1983 Andrew had just ended a six-year gay relationship and was working as a steward for Continental Airlines when he noticed a blue spot on his ankle. He thought nothing of it at the time. Only later when he began to suffer intense tiredness and night sweats — classic symptoms of AIDS — did he begin to fear the worst. By the end of the year, he had lost more than 14 lb (6.4 kg) in weight and was suffering severe pain from a rare form of cancer called Burkitt's lymphoma. He was hospitalized but made a good recovery, his family staying by his bed all the time.

When he returned home, Andrew was still weak and helpless. Nevertheless, he was welcomed, although there were problems — for instance when an extended visit from a young niece and nephew had to be cut short because their father feared they might get AIDS. As Andrew said in an interview in *Newsweek*, it made him feel 'like a piece of crawling crud that no one could touch'.

These slights were minor compared to the ones suffered by 32-year-old construction worker Robert. He began to develop severe shortness of breath which turned into pneumonia, caused by AIDS. He was too weak to work or to take care of himself. Robert was alone and without money, his parents were dead and he was estranged from his brothers. Even his former lover rejected him and threw him out of his apartment, fearing that he might otherwise contract AIDS.

When Robert's plight was publicized in *The Baltimore Sun*, it caused a furore. Several 'foster' families came forward to provide shelter. But in the end, their kindly intentions came to nothing. One family refused to have him for more than a weekend because they said he was spilling blood on sheets, and another had to give up when they received threatening phone calls and had their car vandalized. When he was last interviewed, Robert was in hospital, suffering from severe pneumonia, only conscious for brief periods and scarcely strong enough to utter more than a few words.

These stories, and many similar tragedies, were by now becoming all too familar. But the story that grabbed more headlines and which featured on more magazine covers (including *Life*), was that of a young couple living in a quiet rural area of the US. Pat is a haemophiliac and contracted AIDS after being treated with contaminated factor VIII. Tragically, Pat was unaware of his condition and passed on the disease to his wife, Lauren. She was pregnant, and their baby son Dwight was subsequently born suffering from AIDS as well. The only member of the family untouched by the virus's dreadful effects was Pat's young daughter, Nicole. The thought that their young son was doomed to die so soon after birth was a final bitter twist to the family's awful story. 'I grew up with haemophilia and I said that all the things that I couldn't do, my son would be able to. He would make up for both of us', says Pat. 'But now my boy is going to die'.

By this time, the psychological effect on the gay community in the US was becoming a serious problem in its own right. As the owner of one San Francisco bath-house put it: 'There is a cloud, a fog that hangs over our heads constantly. You cannot go into a bar where everyone is not talking about AIDS'. There were also signs of a disturbing reaction from the general public. After a few years of relative freedom from prejudice, and of being allowed to carry on with open relationships, homosexuals began to suffer serious victimization again. Some were sacked, others were evicted from their apartments. Technicians on a New York television station refused to work in a studio in which an AIDS victim was being interviewed, while many gays found they were being shouted at, spat at, or punched in the street. As one gay put it: 'For fifteen years, we all had a party. It was so good that you couldn't help thinking how it was going to end'.

By mid-1982, he had his answer. It was ending in tragedy. One gay couple in New York simply chose a suicide pact. On learning that he was dying of AIDS, 33-year-old Charles, and his lover, 44-year-old Gilbert, went on a spending spree, drank a last bottle of expensive wine, and then flung themselves from the balcony of their flat, tied together by a silk sash.

The crisis worsened when AIDS began to spread through US jails. One of the worst affected was Sing Sing, near New York (where 135 prisoners were to die of AIDS within four years). With grimly ironic humour, prisoners gave the name 'Death Row' to the AIDS unit in the hospital there. In prisons, infections are caused mainly by intravenous drug use among prisoners. Those afflicted with AIDS suffer particularly severe deprivation. Locked in cells, for 24 hours a day, they have little to do but to dwell on their condition. Nor can they expect sympathetic treatment from guards. One prisoner in Sing Sing recalls an officer who dressed up in a gown and mask and threatened to kill prisoners with a piece of lead piping if they came near him. Another promised to shoot inmates. Guards wanted rid of them and prisoners were desperate for release. But the public outside was equally adamant that affected prisoners should be kept locked up. As a result, by 1985 only one of Sing Sing's AIDS victims ever managed to get parole, so he could be left to die in freedom.

Such tragedies were no longer being confined to the US, however. In 1982, the first, inevitable evidence of AIDS' spread to other continents was discovered. Cases were reported from several areas of the world. Some of these occurred — in Europe and Japan for instance — as a result of dependence on the US for supplies of factor VIII for haemophiliacs. Others occurred when gays and drug addicts returned from holidays and business trips to the US.

One of the first cases to be discovered in Britain was that of Terrence Higgins, a 37-year-old homosexual. (His name has subsequently been dedicated to the UK's first AIDS victims support group, the Terrence Higgins Trust.) His symptoms were classic indications of AIDS. They began with feelings of malaise, sickness, night sweats and shivering. Later they included chronic diarrhoea, incontinence and then delirium. Terrence was taken to hospital suffering from pneumonia. At times he could not even recognize friends and family who had come to see him.

Doctors at St Thomas's Hospital, London managed to cure Terrence's pneumonia by treating him with powerful drugs. But shortly afterwards, he contracted a new infection, toxoplasmosis. Caused by a ubiquitous one-celled creature called a protozoan, toxoplasmosis can be a deadly infection that affects both the brain and lungs. Normally the body's powerful immune defences can mop up the offending protozoa. Without these defences, Terrence was powerless to resist their attack. On 4 July, 1982, he died. AIDS had arrived in Britain.

Very shortly, the same tragedies which had struck in the US were being repeated in Britain. One victim is Chris, of West London, who was only nineteen when he was first diagnosed as having AIDS. He told his story on the BBC television programme, *Panorama.*

'I was getting very fatigued and my weight went down from nine to seven stone. It was gradual and I didn't really notice anything unusual at first.' Chris's body temperature then began to rise dramatically during sleep, causing night sweats. 'By morning, my bed would be drenched', he recalls. Later Chris contracted pneumonia, although his doctor did not recognize which variety at first. 'I was given the wrong sort of antibiotics and I collapsed', says Chris. He has subsequently responded well to treatments, and is now in reasonable health, using his Buddhist beliefs as a source of strength. Nevertheless, he has suffered. 'I have gone through a lot of pain. But the real problem is the fear of the unknown.'

Chris's story is a relatively encouraging one. Other tales have been less reassuring, like the case of Richard. His story is a horrifying compilation of medical complacency and ineptness which revealed that in 1983 some areas of the health service were still not ready to cope with AIDS, two years after cases had first been reported to them. Richard and his family's ordeal began in later 1983 when Richard, an Oxford scholar and art historian, began to develop swellings and boils whenever he cut himself shaving. 'In the end, his face was covered in suppurating sores', recalls his sister Ruth. These boils were clear signals that Richard's immune system was breaking down under the onslaught of the AIDS virus.

Richard had never made any secret of his homosexuality. His family certainly knew. Yet diagnosis of his condition completely escaped Richard's family practice. 'He visited them several times, but they didn't even give him antibiotics, although his symptoms were alarming', adds Ruth. In the end Richard stopped asking for treatment, complaining that he was being made to feel a hypochondriac, although by this time he was also suffering from fever, glandular swellings, chest and throat infections and fatigue

By spring 1984, Richard had been transformed from a dynamic young man who did regular weight training, French translation work and art history research, into a painfully thin, depressed and lethargic invalid who spent much of his time asleep on couches in the family's elegant North London apartment. 'His whole personality changed', says his mother. 'He became very insecure and depressed. Not knowing what was wrong got him down all the more'. Ruth adds: 'Obviously we thought he might have AIDS but you do not dwell on the idea that such a rare disease might be affecting someone you love'. By October 1984,

Richard's condition had seriously deteriorated. In fact, he was suffering from pneumonia, a severe fungal infection of the mouth, and a Kaposi's tumour of the palate. Diagnoses of these conditions would have been sure signs that Richard had AIDS, but almost unbelievably his doctors failed to spot any of them.

Then Richard's temperature suddenly soared to 104° F (40° C). He was taken to hospital where he was immediately put in an isolation ward and his visitors were required to wear masks. When his mother asked the reason for such measures, she was told by the consultant that Richard had pneumonia and AIDS 'which should come as no surprise given his lifestyle.' As she put it: 'We knew Richard was gay and accepted it. However, I might not have known and that would have come as another shock. I was also told nothing about the disease or its prognosis. Later, when I told the consultant I was worried that my other son Robert, who shared a bathroom with Richard, might get AIDS, he giggled and said: "Not unless he has been up to the same shenanigans and has been mixing with the same company." That was the level of his counselling.'

At 2 a.m. the next morning, the ward sister phoned and told the family that Richard was dead. 'We arranged for his coffin to be brought home for two days for friends to see him before his funeral. On the day he was due, I got a hysterical phone call from the undertaker who accused me of deceit and of trying to infect his staff because I had not said Richard had AIDS. He ended up screaming down the phone at me. Eventually, Richard was delivered in the plastic bag in which he left the hospital and inside a sealed coffin. He was treated all the time like a carrier of the Black Death.'

The story of Richard is a sorry one. His GP failed totally to diagnose a well-described and very serious illness. This would not have saved Richard's life but could have prolonged it, perhaps to give him time to see his father and grandmother in Australia. In addition, his consultant was uncaring and tactless to say the least, while his undertakers reacted with brutal disregard for the feelings of a grieving family. 'It is right to treat AIDS with alarm', admits Ruth, 'but not with hysteria and feelings of retribution that have been our experiences'.

In fact, hysteria and retribution were to become all-too-common experiences for many AIDS victims and their families. Fortunately, there were others whose predicaments were treated more compassionately. The story of Arthur illustrates both sides — the unrelenting and the humane.

In December, 1984, Arthur was diagnosed as having PCP. He was placed in a special isolation ward at London's Charing Cross Hospital where he was treated with powerful antibiotics that cured him of his pneumonia. A homesexual with a circle of about a dozen causal friends who were his regular lovers, 45-year-old Arthur now acknowledges that he should have been very careful about his sexual partners but was not. 'I knew about AIDS. You couldn't miss hearing about it by then. I just didn't accept that I was in danger. I should have done but I believed it couldn't happen to me. If I had thought about it, I would have realized I was among those most at risk. The only answer would have been to give up my lifestyle. I was enjoying myself too much at that time to want to do that. So I just didn't think about AIDS.'

Arthur was cured of his pneumonia but still found his health impaired. 'I was drained. I used to come home, switch on the TV and sit there all evening until it was bedtime.' A civil servant working at London's Wormwood Scrubs prison, Arthur had not attempted to conceal his homosexuality from his colleagues. 'However, when I was first ill, I covered things up by saying I had pneumonia. I didn't mention AIDS.' But later, Arthur began to suffer severe bouts of fever. He was hospitalized in February — in the week that British newspapers embarked on their first full wave of AIDS hysteria. The triggering event was the death, from AIDS, of Chelmsford prison chaplain Greg

Richard. 'Papers began publishing all sorts of sensational things. They also began describing details of the symptoms of AIDS', adds Arthur. 'It was not long before someone at work realized I had those symptoms.'

A television news team visiting Wormwood Scrubs was told of Arthur's condition and of his confinement at Charing Cross hospital. Within hours, the hospital was besieged by TV camera teams and newspaper reporters.

> The hospital administrator came into my room. He told me that the place was virtually surrounded by the Press and that he had released a statement admitting that a 45-year-old civilian worker from Wormwood Scrubs had been admitted to Charing Cross with suspected AIDS. I couldn't believe it. I knew people would easily have identified me from that description.
>
> For the first time since I was diagnosed as having AIDS, I broke down and cried. I was so angry and frustrated.

Arthur phoned his ex-lover to warn him about the impending publicity and to ask him to phone his mother and four children (from his old marriage).

> He told me I was too late. I had already been on the BBC News.
>
> I watched the next bulletin. I was stunned. I had pushed the miners' national strike into third place. Only the outcome of a big security trial came before my story. The announcer gave my age and place of work and said I had been taken to Charing Cross 'suffering from AIDS.' Only in later bulletins was that changed to 'suspected AIDS'.
>
> It was incredible. From the sensational way they described things, you would have thought I was a threat to the nation's health, not a man who was ill and alone.

There was worse to follow. The next day, Britain's more lurid Sunday newspapers followed up his story. The *Sunday People* said Arthur (though they did not name him) was suffering from the gay plague and that the news had 'shocked prison authorities and staff who weren't told why he was on sick leave'.

These stories only increased Arthur's isolation. He attempted to return to work — but was suspended on full pay, pending an enquiry, because of the publicity. 'That really infuriated me. The Home Office, which runs the prison service, had already announced that it was safe to work with people who had AIDS. Yet they wouldn't let me go back.' However, after several weeks off work, Arthur was allowed to return. His story then took a happier turn:

> The weekend before my return date, several colleagues phoned and asked if I wanted to meet them outside work, so I could walk through the prison gates with them for moral support. I was very grateful but decided I must do it myself — though I was nervous. There had been all sorts of stories published about AIDS sufferers who were shunned and insulted at work. When I got to the prison gate, the guard just looked at me, smiled and said: 'Welcome back, Arthur'. It was as simple and pleasant as that.

On his desk, Arthur found a bottle of champagne and a greeting card signed by his colleagues. 'Everyone treated me wonderfully. Only one woman spoiled things by insisting on wearing rubber gloves when she was handling objects that I had touched. She soon realized she was being silly and stopped, however.'

Arthur's experiences were ultimately reassuring, although his treatment by television and newspapers, which besieged his hospital and sensationalized his condition, has left him with bitter views about the Press. 'I loathe the tabloid papers for their treatment of my predicament and those of other AIDS patients. Most of their stories have just been vicious lies.' There are now many others who share that view.

3

'Abnormal, Unnatural and Evil'

In early 1985, a young female nurse at a British hospital accidently injected herself with blood taken from an AIDS patient. She developed a flu-like reaction and then recovered. Subsequent tests revealed she was carrying the virus HTLV3/LAV in her blood. It was an unfortunate incident, although it is the only known case in the world in which the virus responsible for AIDS has definitely been picked up accidentally by a health worker in the course of his or her duties. She has been treated in a markedly different way to health workers who have picked up the disease in other ways, however. Indeed, these cases illustrate a clear and dangerous disparity that has developed in attitudes towards the disease. In another case, a male gay nurse picked up the virus from a lover while off duty. He was sacked as a health risk to patients. The nurse who accidentally injected herself was allowed to continue working at her hospital.

'What is the difference?', asks Les Lattner, of the Terrence Higgins Trust. 'If carrying the AIDS virus is a health risk, both should surely have lost their jobs. If carrying the virus is not a health risk — as scientists say — then neither should have lost their posts. The fact that one did, and the other did not, shows that hospital authorities were really passing judgement on the lifestyles of the two nurses. The decisions that were made had nothing to do with their states of health.'

The case is unfortunate, although it is certainly not the worst example of discrimination to come to light as AIDS has gained greater notoriety. Indeed, since the start of the epidemic, the public has frequently reacted with hysteria, and has treated many homosexuals — affected or unaffected — as lepers. Yet gays are not a threat to the public. In fact, the real risks come from ignorance about the spread of the AIDS virus to bridging groups. These are made up of people who have had intimate contacts with members of risk groups, such as gays and drug addicts, and who have now picked up the virus. They may soon begin to pass on AIDS to the general population — not, of course, by touching, but by sexual contact.

It is a situation that should be treated with alarm, but not with hysteria. Unfortunately, those most needed to help in the hunt for these bridging group members are the ones who are being most alienated because they are suffering the worst victimization. Sometimes, this discrimination is overt, even violent. At other times it is subtle. The language of newspapers is an example of the latter. Women, children and haemophiliacs are invariably labelled 'innocent' victims. The adjective is never used to describe homosexuals. A clear distinction is made this way — that gays are guilty and deserve their fate, while others are innocent. A new hierarchy of blame has been created by the media.

It is a tendency that now worries many gay rights activists. 'The media is concentrating on areas where there is prejudice already. We are seeing a new legitimizing of that prejudice', states Lorraine Trenchard, of Gays in Broadcasting. Many newspapermen agree: 'Fleet Street does not like homosexuality', admitted former *Daily Star* editor, Derek Jamieson, on a special edition of the BBC TV programme, *Open Space*, which was devoted to the Press's treatment of AIDS. 'They think it is abnormal, unnatural and evil because it is wrong.' An epidemic of a disease that strikes at gays is therefore considered to be fair game for sensationalism.

Indeed, from the start most newspapers have treated AIDS as if it is a contagious disease and have constantly questioned scientists and doctors' continual assurances that it is not. At the same time, papers have ignored the real risks. By seeing AIDS as a 'gay plague' and not as a general sexually transmitted disease that can affect men and women, they have misled the public.

A particularly lurid example of this sensationalism appeared on the front page of *The Sunday People* — on the same day that it published its version of Arthur's story and of his confinement at Charing Cross Hospital. Under the claim 'World Exclusive', the paper printed the giant headline 'Scandal of AIDS cover-up on QE2'. The story underneath alleged that passengers and crew on the Cunard liner had been deceived by an 'astounding cover-up'. The 'deception' involved a passenger who was suffering from 'the terrifying gay plague', AIDS. Cunard had not announced this fact, it was 'revealed'. The article then quoted passengers who, on being told there had been an AIDS sufferer in their midst, claimed that their lives had been put at risk. The story implied they were justified in their fears. They were not, of course. Only sexual intercourse with the man — 'a homosexual millionaire who was also suffering from cancer' — could have put them at risk, or if an exchange of blood had taken place. Such fates were unlikely to befall heterosexual passengers on a luxury liner, to say the least — though *The Sunday People* never mentioned this point.

Of course, sensation and prejudice have not been limited to tabloid newspapers when debating AIDS. In one astonishing leader on the disease which was published by *The Times* on 21 November 1984, it was stated that: 'AIDS horrifies not only because of the prognosis for its victims. The infection's origins and means of propagation excites repugnance, moral and physical, at promiscuous male homosexuality.' To be so attacked in a quality newspaper which also implied that AIDS was 'some sort of retribution', only served to increase the isolation of Britain's homosexuals. However, such bigotry was topped by *The Daily Mail* on 24 December 1985. Commenting on the last photograph taken of actor Rock Hudson, AIDS' most famous victim to date, it described his features as 'dissipated, corrupt, and decadent'.

Professor Michael Adler, a leading AIDS clinician and researcher based at the Middlesex Hospital, London, describes such reporting as 'witch-hunting and soap box moralizing'. Richard Wells, an adviser at the Royal College of Nursing, puts it more strongly: 'I think every newspaper should now be forced to carry a government health warning', he says.

But the media has not been alone in its hounding of homosexuals as AIDS has spread. Senior White House adviser Pat Buchanan stunned gays throughout the United States by announcing: 'Poor homosexuals. They have declared war on nature and now nature is exacting an awful retribution.' Nor did homosexuals appreciate the utterances of Louie Welch, candidate for the mayor of Houston, during election hustings in October 1985. Unaware that his microphone had been turned on just before a television interview, he announced that the best way to halt AIDS' spread would be to 'shoot the queers'. Later Welch claimed he had just been 'horsing around' and that his remark had been just a joke. Most gays in his audience thought it decidedly unfunny, however. Nor were they amused by the spread of other AIDS 'jokes', such as car stickers which claim that 'AIDS is a gift of the fairies' and which urge other motorists to 'Help Stamp Out AIDS — Run Down a Queer'.

AIDS even became a national election issue in Australia in 1984, when thirteen people died after being given blood contaminated with the virus. The right-wing Australian National Party blamed the Labour government for encouraging homosexuality as 'a normal relationship' while newspapers carried banner headlines about the hunt for remaining bottles of infected blood. Prime Minister Bob Hawke held an 'AIDS summit' with senior medical advisers and homosexuals were told they would be prosecuted if they were caught donating blood. (An AIDS blood test was still not available then.)

Even the medical profession has sometimes reacted in questionable ways. In Britain, doctors refused to carry out autopsies on two homosexuals because they had heard rumours that the two gays had suffered from AIDS. At the inquest, one of the doctors claimed forensic staff could have been infected during the autopsy. But Westminster coroner Dr Paul Knapman was not impressed. 'If an outbreak of mass hysteria breaks out among the medical profession, how can we expect the rest of the country to behave?', he asked.

Indeed, on both sides of the Atlantic, people have begun to react in peculiar, and frightening, ways to the disease. In Atlanta, one man was seen dousing his backyard with powerful insecticide lest mosquitos bite guests at his gay neighbour's barbecue and then carry the AIDS virus to him. Other cases were even more astonishing. Delta Airlines refused to carry AIDS victims until gay rights activists forced a reversal of this decision; cleaners at a Swansea theatre, venue for a play featuring gay actors, demanded special protective clothing for their work; churches were told by parishioners that they would not take communion for fear of picking up AIDS from chalices; and firemen were advised by their union not to give the kiss of life.

In the US, as Trevor Fishlock, *The Times* correspondent in New York, reported — the fear of AIDS became as much a phenomenon as AIDS itself. In one despatch he told of a series of astonishing incidents that were typical of a wave of over-reaction that swept the country. In one case, a doctor began to badger health authorities in Boston in a bid to get AIDS victims sent to a former leper colony on an island off Massachusetts. In another incident, an AIDS virus carrier was charged with trying to murder four policemen by trying to spit at them! Fishlock reported thus:

In many minds, AIDS has taken on the terrifying characteristics of a plague. People have even become nervous about eating in restaurants with homosexual staff. A couple visiting New Orleans reported being so nervous of eating out that they lived off tinned food in their hotel room.

Yet experts say people stand a greater chance of being struck by lightning than by AIDS. But many people do not trust experts and there is a strong feeling of 'better safe than sorry' in their minds.

In Hollywood, AIDS was an obsession among film producers and actors, even before the death of Hudson. Stars, such as Bo Derek, have insisted that their co-stars sign contracts in which they affirm that they do not carry the AIDS virus. In this way, it is hoped that a screen kiss will not pass on the dreaded disease.

Much of California has been gripped by similar panics. By 1985, powerful black markets were established for drugs, such as isoprinosine and ribavarin, following reports that they had alleviated some victims' conditions. These are not licensed in the US, but are freely and cheaply available from pharmacists in nearby Mexico and have been imported illegally to California in large amounts.

Gays themselves have sometimes reacted in puzzling ways. In America, some have set up groups with sensible motives, such as Orgiasts Anonymous, an organisation that attempts to persuade gays not to have sex with strangers who might otherwise give them AIDS. Others have gone to opposite extremes, however. One such group is Homosexuals Intrangisent. Its aim is to encourage promiscuous gays to continue in their former ways, despite the dangers of contracting AIDS in the process. As Les Lattner says: 'Some gays still like to cruise. The thought that their next pick-up might be the one to give them AIDS provides them with a real turn on.'

Even Cold War conspiracy theories have been put forward to account for the appearance and spread of AIDS. *The Literary Gazette*, the weekly magazine of the Soviet Writer's Union, has accused the CIA and the Pentagon of unleashing the virus, which it suggested was the by-product of a military experiment that had gone disastrously wrong. For its part, the extreme right-wing US journal, *Executive Intelligence Review*, has blamed the entire epidemic on similar sorts of experiments by Soviet military scientists.

In the midst of such lunacy, citizens could be forgiven for being muddled in their reactions to AIDS. Nevertheless, some of their responses have been disturbing. A poll published by *The Los Angeles Times* in December 1985 revealed that of 2,308 people interviewed, 50 per cent favoured the quarantining of AIDS victims, 48 per cent said they should be given special identification tags; and 15 per cent called for them to be tattoed.

These reactions reveal a dangerous tendency of thinking of AIDS as an external threat. It is not, though it is possible to understand why people think this. As one AIDS counsellor, Christopher Spence, says:

> AIDS impinges on our lives in the very places where we tend to be numb already and often via the graphic horror stories which make hot journalism. It is therefore hardly surprising that AIDS is so often resisted as an issue relevant to everyone and is sometimes dismissed altogether as the penalty of fast-lane living. The truth is that AIDS profoundly affects us all — men, women and children.

Writing in a pamphlet produced by the Terrence Higgins Trust, he adds:

> Any issue affecting people at the level of life and death is an issue for everyone. Any issue housing the excuse for increased mistreatment of a particular group within society is an issue for everyone. And any issue raising questions of sexual practice, as AIDS does, is undoubtedly an issue for everyone.

But the popular support for extreme containment measures which was revealed in the Los Angeles poll now seriously worries many counsellors who are trying to help victims and who are attempting to find ways to halt the spread of the disease. Counsellors fear that increased discrimination will alienate gays when they are most needed to help contain the AIDS epidemic. The real risks lie elsewhere, they say. Pressure to segregate homosexuals (and possibly other members of risk groups) may also prove to be dangerously counterproductive. Already, signs are developing that AIDS victims and virus carriers may soon be driven underground.

This problem is illustrated by Jonathan Grimshaw, of Body Positive. His group exists to help carriers of the AIDS virus (of whom at least one in ten will develop the full syndrome, say scientists). 'When I was first told that I was carrying the virus, I was shattered. It was not just the anxiety. It was the tremendous feeling of isolation. A barrier was thrown up between me and the rest of the world'. Jonathan's experiences reveal the power of that sort of barrier. 'I was devastated. My life was thrown into upheaval. I knew I could not have any more late nights, alcohol or other pleasures to which I was accustomed in case I triggered a full attack of AIDS'. Other virus carriers have suffered rejection and vilification.

These are some of the factors that put pressure on carriers, strengthening the barriers between them and the rest of society. And with stronger and stronger barriers erected around them, homosexuals (and others perceived as being risks) will be less and less likely to co-operate with the authorities in their attempts to trace carriers and victims. Another reason for gays' reluctance to co-operate with medical authorities is explained by Tony Whitehead, of the Terrence Higgins Trust. 'The British government says it needs the co-operation of gays to fight the spread of AIDS. But why should we co-operate with them? The government has done absolutely nothing for us in the past. Why should we be expected to co-operate now?'

There are other problems. 'If homosexuals — who are still the main group affected by AIDS after all — are increasingly victimized and treated as lepers, they may well not come forward for testing', adds Dr David Miller, of St Mary's Hospital, London:

It may do them little good if they do. They may only be victimized all the more if it is found that they are virus positive. The same goes for the tracing of homosexual contacts. It is bad enough at present. There is still a great stigma attached to homosexuality. Many people still do not admit to it. There are certainly many respectable, married businessmen who are secretly homosexual. These bisexuals are usually terrified that someone might reveal their homosexual tendencies.

That terror will only increase, the more that gays are accused of being health dangers. The homosexual partners of these 'respectable' bisexuals will be under even greater pressure not to name them as contacts — even if one of them is found to be carrying the AIDS virus. Yet these bisexuals are the very ones that medical authorities want to trace. They may pass the virus on to their wives, or to other homosexual contacts, after all. They are the bridging groups. The ones who might spread the disease into the general population.

This is where the real danger of the spread of AIDS lies. It does not come from being close to infected gays, but from having intimate relations with seemingly innocuous, and apparently uninfected, people — the members of the bridging groups of prostitutes, bisexuals, partners of haemophiliacs and drug addicts. They are the ones who may carry the disease out of high risk groups into the general population.

In the case of bisexuals, the extent of the problem can be appreciated when it is realized that at least 2 per cent of married men are thought to be predominantly homosexual and that as many as 50 per cent of all men may have had overt homosexual experiences at some point in their lives. In Britain, a total of 13 million men are covered by that definition, though few would admit it. And they are only one of several bridging groups that threaten to spread AIDS.

Indeed, the problem appears already to be worryingly well-developed — as is illustrated in the elegant Georgian surroundings of Scotland's capital, Edinburgh. Away from the main tourist attractions, there is another Edinburgh, a city of back streets and apartments where there are drug users who share syringes and inject heroin. These people are found in all major towns of the West today and are an extremely worrying aspect of the bridging group problem. 'A lot of the people really just don't care less,' said Alex, a young Edinburgh heroin user on the Thames Television *TV Eye* programme, 'AIDS and You', screened in November, 1985. 'I've seen people drop needles in puddles and pick them up, just washing them out and using them — as long as they got their shot. A lot of the time, I just shared somebody else's needle, I was so desperate to get the heroin into myself.'

This casual abuse of syringes has reaped a bitter harvest for the young drug users of the city — one that reveals that AIDS may have already penetrated deeply into parts of the heterosexual population. A study by University of Edinburgh researchers, carried out in late 1985, showed that 38 per cent of the drug users who were tested were carrying the AIDS virus in their blood.

'This was both males and females', said one of the doctors, John Pleutherer. 'If you'd asked me beforehand, I would have said that perhaps 5 or 6 per cent might have been infected. However, after checking and re-checking, we were left with this figure of 38 per cent.' It is an alarming statistic. It means that in addition to dealing with drug addiction, doctors must now cope with AIDS' spread among these addicts as well. But what really worries medical authorities is the threat these infected people pose to unsuspecting members of the public. The danger could come from the outwardly respectable person who only shoots heroin at weekends, for instance. Or it could come from the girl who sleeps with her boyfriend unaware that he takes drugs and is infected. As AIDS takes months, sometimes years, to manifest itself, she could become infected herself and could even begin to spread the virus to others before discovering she was carrying HTLV3/LAV in her blood.

In other parts of Britain, the spread of AIDS virus among drug takers still seems to be relatively low. However, in other countries, it has already reached dramatic levels. By late 1985, the prevalence was thought to be about 35 per cent among users in Switzerland and Spain, while one study in New York found that 87 per cent of addicts carried the AIDS virus.

Among haemophiliacs a similar frightening increase in AIDS infections has taken place. In one survey by Dr Richard Tedder, of the Middlesex Hosptial, London, it was discovered that the first infections had occurred in 1980 among patients who had been treated with commerical factor VIII concentrates from the US. By 1981, 50 per cent were carrying antibodies to the AIDS virus (which showed they had been infected). The figure rose to 64 per cent by 1982 and to 66 per cent by 1983. These figures correspond closely with the results of similar studies of haemophiliacs in Denmark and the US where prevalence rates of 64 and 72 per cent were found respectively.

By 1985, Dr Brian Colvin, director of the London Hospital's haemophilia centre, estimated that in Britain between 70 and 90 per cent of severe haemophilia sufferers — who take most factor VIII injections — had been infected with the AIDS virus. As Dr Tedder commented, these widespread infections are 'laying down a heritage of disease for the future. The problem is not preventing the virus getting into the community — it is there already — but in being able to cope with it.'

Doctors also acknowledged there was a risk of contracting AIDS during standard blood transfusions, although this was considered to be extremely low. For instance, in 1985, a 21-month-old baby died of AIDS in Britain after the child was given transfusions of contaminated blood during a heart operation in the US. In general, it was estimated that one case of AIDS occurs for every quarter of a million transfusions that were carried out in the US. However, for those who were suffering from leukaemia or who required heart surgery, and therefore need large amounts of blood, possibly from many donors, the risk was greater. As a result, blood banks in the US, the American Red Cross and some British doctors recommended that patients expecting surgery should donate their own blood in anticipation of its use during their operations. However, the susequent introduction of heat treatment of factor VIII and the screening of donors have made blood supplies much safer.

The degree to which the last remaining bridging group — prostitutes — is infected is not so well documented, although evidence suggests that in many cities there are pockets of high AIDS virus prevalence among prostitutes. In many central African cities, such as Nairobi and Kigali (the capital of Rwanda) there are certainly large numbers of prostitutes who are infected. Western cities, including New York and Vienna, are also thought to have become problem areas. The chances of picking up the AIDS virus this way is considered to be serious by doctors such as John Harris, a London consultant. He has warned businessmen travelling abroad to take care about sleeping with prostitutes: 'I think there is now a serious risk that businessmen can pick up AIDS and pass it on after travelling abroad', he told a conference on sexually transmitted diseases in Brighton.

It is now clear that bridging groups are the key to the spread of AIDS. However, it is still not known what is the exact degree of danger posed by them. Men and women can infect each other — but how easily? It has been established that men can infect women. Haemophiliacs, like Pat, have passed on the virus to their wives, for instance, and so have drug addicts. As HTLV3/LAV is carried in semen, it is possible to understand how they might infect women through sexual intercourse. But it has not been established exactly how women could infect men by the same route, although this certainly can occur.

'The exact mode of sexual transmission of the AIDS virus is still not perfectly understood at present', admits Dr Tony

Pinching. 'In Africa, almost as many women as men are infected — and that suggests the virus is passing fairly easily between them. However, in the West, similar evidence is generally anecdotal. I take these stories seriously, however. Today's anecdotes are tomorrow's epidemiology.' The ease with which HTLV3/LAV passes from women to men may ultimately determine the rate at which the general population succumbs to AIDS. If it does not pass very easily between them, increases in infections will be slow. If it does pass easily, then AIDS may spread with devastating rapidity.

At present, there is disagreement among scientists about the likely rate of this spread. Dr Victor Daniels, a UK observer of the disease, and the UK medical director of an international pharmaceutical company, believes the failure of AIDS to move widely into the community is striking. He points out that in one US study, only two wives of haemophiliacs were found to be HTLV3/LAV positive. 'There is however still the worrying possiblity of heterosexual spread of the disease outside the usual risk groups', he admits.

Evidence that supports the prospect of heterosexual spread comes from scientists such as Dr Robert Redfield, of the US Army's Walter Reed Hospital, who reported at an international medical conference in Atlanta in 1985 that of 41 AIDS patients examined at a Washington hospital, nearly a third had had no contact with any members of high risk groups, such as homosexuals or drug addicts. The common factor in their lifestyles was heterosexual sex with a very large number of partners — more than 100 — over the previous five years. Often these partners were prostitutes. Such studies have so alarmed US military officials that they have begun to broadcast special radio warnings to US troops stationed in Europe to tell them that prostitutes in some cities may be harbouring the AIDS virus and could pass it on to them during sexual intercourse.

Christopher Spence also believes the disease can be

spread between women and men. Its high prevalence among homosexuals in the US and Europe can be understood because gays have little direct contact with heterosexuals, he says. So far, there has simply not been enough time for the virus to move out of these groups into the general population. 'If such a disease is introduced into a group which has sexual contact primarily with other members of that group, then it will initially show up most often within that group, as is the case with gay men', he states.

This interpretation is shared by Professor Julian Peto, of London's Institute of Cancer Research. 'If you look at the numbers of heterosexuals outside high risk groups and who are now contracting AIDS, then they appear to be very low. In fact, cases are just about at the same level as was found among homosexuals when AIDS was first discovered', he says. 'Since then there has been a huge multiplication in numbers of gays going down with the disease. The evidence suggests the same thing will happen in the general population.'

AIDS was discovered in 1981. By 1985, 20,000 cases had been found in a total of 73 countries, the World Health Organization announced in December 1985. It also revealed that numbers were doubling every eight or nine months. However, most doctors and scientists think that this is a very conservative estimate and that it hides a huge number of cases that have developed in Africa. 'I really think AIDS is going to be the worst thing in the public health domain for many decades,' says Professor Peto:

> It will prove to be more devastating than the flu epidemics which occurred at the beginning of the century, for instance. Those killed millions of people, but at least the virus responsible came and went. The AIDS virus seems to stay in the body for a very long time. The dreadful feature about AIDS is that it doesn't matter what level it is finally contained at, it will be with us forever. It is going to be an epidemic of appalling dimensions for the forseeable future, no matter what control measures are taken.

This cataclysmic interpretation is echoed in the words of Dr Pinching:

I think AIDS is the most serious health problem we have faced this century. It is already affecting the developed world and parts of the developing world — and if we do not rise to the challenge of its spread, it will get worse and worse. In ten years, it will be endemic. We will have to live with AIDS as a perpetual risk to our healths and lives. Then people will no longer make the mistake of only associating the disease with a particular type of lifestyle which they consider to be foreign and strange. We will no longer look upon AIDS with the voyeurism with which we do today and see it as someone else's problem. By then it will touch upon all our lives.

4

The French Connection

Dr Robert Gallo is one of America's most distinguished and renowned scientists. Based at the National Cancer Institutes in Washington, the 48-year-old biologist has had a brilliant career that was capped in 1978 by his discovery of one of the first viruses known to cause cancers in humans. His impact on the study of AIDS has been equally profound. It has also been extraordinarily controversial.

'Gallo is very gifted', says one of Britain's leading AIDS researchers. 'He is also thin-skinned, ambitious and vain. It has caused a lot of conflict.' The hostilities stem from the intense rivalry that has sprung up between Gallo and his French counterparts, who are led by Dr Luc Montagnier and are based at the Pasteur Institute in Paris. There, scientists have also battled to pinpoint the virus responsible for AIDS.

Both teams' efforts have been classic scientific stories of false leads, disappointments, setbacks, amazing luck, endless drudgery, and instinctive inspiration. They have also been marked by bitter, often distasteful, personal battles that have eventually resulted in the French accusing Gallo of scientific misconduct. As the US science journal *Discover* put it: 'It is a story of arrogance, scientific élitism and strong egos in an intense, unfriendly competition that many observers believe may have hampered the exchange of vital data.'

Nor have the French gone without their share of criticism. The same British scientist who passed comment on Gallo, adds: 'He may have his faults but they are openly displayed. Gallo wears his personality on his sleeve. Montagnier is more assured and polite in public, but he is also more cunning in private.' The story of their battle begins in 1982 when Gallo — after more than a decade of brilliant achievements in cell biology, molecular biology and virology — decided to join the search for the virus that was beginning to devastate so many different groups of Americans. An intense and ambitious competitor, Gallo is once alleged to have said that 'I want to be something better than the best I have ever seen'. Gallo gave himself two years to complete his self-appointed task. 'The fact that he set himself such a goal is in itself a credit to Gallo', says Dr Dalgleish. 'Many other scientists with his record might have been tempted to give up and rest on their reputations. He did not.'

At that time, Gallo's scientific reputation rested principally on his discovery of a type of virus, called a *retrovirus*, which causes a form of leukaemia in people. Scientists had never before traced retroviruses to diseases in humans, though they had linked them to illnesses in animals. To understand the actions of retroviruses and, for that matter all other types of virus, we have to look closely at the structure of our bodies. We are made up of millions of individual cells which combine to form skin, bones, eyes, and other organs. The growth and development of these cells are controlled by tiny packets of material called DNA (deoxyribonucleic acid) which lie at the centres of all cells.

Although each DNA packet — which is called a chromosome — is extremely small and can only be seen through a microscope, it contains a massive amount of information which determines the characteristics of a cell and ultimately controls the colour of our eyes, height, sex, and countless other features. But when we are infected by viruses, something goes wrong with the behaviour of some of our cells' DNA (or its genes as they are more popularly known). In most cases, our bodies' defences can deal with the attack, but sometimes in serious infections — such as AIDS, rabies, polio or some cancers — the immune system is simply overwhelmed.

A virus is the simplest form of life and attacks by hijacking part of a cell's DNA. Often being little more than a strip of DNA covered in a chemical coat, the virus can insert itself into the host cell's DNA which is then persuaded to make more versions of the virus. These then go on to infect other cells, causing illness. This comandeering form of attack gives rise to the viruses' nickname — the pirates of the cell.

Retroviruses are made of different genetic material called RNA and attack in a slightly different way. They do not directly insert themselves into a host cell's DNA. After entering a cell though its membrane they make a special DNA copy of themselves and this copy is then inserted into the host DNA. As with other viruses, extra copies are then made and these spread round the body.

Scientists had known for a long time that many different types of retrovirus cause illnesses — particularly cancers — in animals. Gallo was one of the first to show they could also result in disease in men and women. Strongly influenced by his own pioneering work, Gallo first speculated that AIDS might be caused by a retrovirus as early as February 1982, at a meeting at the Cold Spring Harbor Laboratories in New York. His ideas were quickly picked up by other scientists, such as Max Essex of the Harvard School of Public Health. The pair had long conversations about the possibility that a retrovirus could be responsible for the new mystery illness which was sweeping the cities and states of the US.

The two scientists were particularly excited by the idea that AIDS might be caused by the same retrovirus that Gallo had originally found in humans. This is called *Human T-cell Leukaemia Virus One,* or HTLV-1 for short. (The '1' is added to distinguish it from a second member of the HTLV family which Gallo had discovered but which he had linked to another form of leukaemia.)*

There was tantalizing evidence to support this theory. For a start, HTLV-1 invades the very cells that are destroyed in AIDS. These are known as T4 cells, or T-helper cells, and are an important part of the body's immune system. There were other clues, however. In cats, the T-cell retrovirus that causes leukaemia also produces a disease with close parallels to AIDS. Affected animals suffer severe immune suppression and often die. Similar effects in humans were also being reported by scientists studying victims of HTLV-1 infections. They too were coming down with opportunistic infections, a bit like those which afflicted AIDS cases. Further evidence was provided from Africa and Haiti. Both have high incidence of HTLV-1 infections and were subsequently found to have large numbers of AIDS cases. As one of Gallo's collaborators, Flossie Wong-Staal, a molecular biologist, stated in an interview in the journal *Science:* 'It looked and smelled like HTLV-1'.

But proving the theory would be a very tricky business because of the effects of AIDS itself. As the disease cripples a vital arm of the immune system, victims are flooded with a range of different viral infections. Among the viruses found in AIDS patients are: cytomegalovirus which can cause infections like meningitis; Epstein-Barr virus, which is often associated with a cancer of the white blood cells; and the herpes simplex virus. Separating these viruses from the one that actually causes AIDS was obviously going to be a difficult task, one that was already causing headaches for other AIDS researchers.

However, Gallo and his team worked hard and produced encouraging results quite quickly. They were particularly excited when they found evidence of a chemical called *reverse transcriptase* in the cells of AIDS patients. Reverse transcriptase is produced when retroviruses make DNA copies of themselves once they are inside infected cells. Despite this success, the National Cancer Institutes team could not grow or directly detect a retrovirus in patients.

Nevertheless, by early 1983 Gallo believed he had assembled enough evidence to show that HTLV-1 was indeed responsible for AIDS. The final confirmation, he believed, was the discovery in several AIDS patients of antibodies in the HTLV-1 virus, or to a virus very like it. Antibodies are special chemicals that are made by the body to block the effects of invading micro-organisms. Each antibody is specially designed to counter a specific microbe. The presence of antibodies which seemed to react to HTLV-1 — or something very like it — was enough to convince Gallo that he was on the right track. He and Essex submitted their findings to the journal *Science* in Spring 1983.

It was an ironic decision, for just as the US scientists were convincing themselves that HTLV-1 was indeed the cause of AIDS, a team of French scientists, led by Dr Montagnier, was coming to a very different conclusion. Calmer, more cautious, and less mercurial than Gallo, Montagnier is nearer to the typical image we have of scientists. He is also close to the stereotype picture of a Frenchman — small, dapper, with a neat moustache and an accent, when speaking English, that is reminiscent Peter Sellers' Inspector Clouseau. Montagnier is also a brilliant researcher.

Working with cells taken from a single patient suffering from lymphadenopathy, a relatively mild gland disorder also caused by the AIDS virus, but which is not usually fatal, Montagnier had also discovered the presence of reverse transcriptase — the footprint of a retrovirus. But where Gallo failed in his attempt to grow the virus in the laboratory, Montagnier succeeded. His team even obtained electron microscope pictures of the viruses as they formed buds on infected cell surfaces prior to their escapes to infect other cells.

Montagnier was convinced that the virus causing AIDS was very different from HTLV-1. It was a retrovirus, admitted Montagnier, but it was quite dissimilar in structure to HTLV-1. He and his team named it lymphadenopathy-associated virus, or LAV. Montagnier wrote up his results for publication in *Science*, which were then, ironically, sent to Gallo to referee. (It is a standard procedure when publishing research results to submit them for independent review prior to publication.) Montagnier's paper duly appeared in *Science* on 20 May 1983 — the very same issue in which Gallo published his paper naming HTLV-1 as the cause of AIDS!

Gallo's results were received with interest and enthusiasm, by some, although others still felt his case for HTLV-1 was weak. Montagnier's paper was greeted with scepticism. This was not particularly surprising. For one thing, Gallo had the greater reputation. More importantly, Montagnier's results were obtained from only one patient. From a single case, it was extremely difficult to tell whether the virus was the real cause of AIDS or was just another opportunistic infection.

Try as he might, Montagnier could not produce the results that would finally convince a cynical scientific world that he had indeed found the culprit responsible for the world's AIDS epidemic. In September 1983, he reported that LAV had been found in the blood of 22 out of a sample of 35 patients suffering from lymphadenopathy. However, as he and his colleagues could not grow their LAV viruses in the quantities needed for a full evaluation of its structure and effects, it was difficult to prove that LAV was indeed the cause of AIDS.

In November 1983, Gallo and his team finally cracked the problem of growing their retrovirus in large enough quantities for proper study. To their surprise, they found that it was not HTLV-1 as they had anticipated, but one with a slightly different structure. Gallo promptly named it HTLV-3.* It was a crucial breakthrough. Developing a method for growing the virus in large amounts allowed the US team to begin developing an AIDS blood test. With plentiful supplies of virus at their disposal, the team could use them to discover which antibodies are produced by the body as it attempts to counter the virus's attack. By identifying these antibodies in other people's blood, it would then be possible to show if they are infected.

The importance of developing a blood test to detect

infection by the AIDS virus cannot be overestimated. Many AIDS virus carriers do not show any outward symptoms and can pass on the disease without realizing they are carriers. An effective test would mean an end to this uncertainty. The team was able to perfect the test very quickly. When used on a group of AIDS patients and on a group of healthy control subjects, it produced remarkable results. Gallo found that more than 90 per cent of the AIDS patients were carrying antibodies while only 1 of his 186 control subjects carried antibodies. These results strongly suggested that Gallo's HTLV-3 was indeed the cause of AIDS. His results were published in the 4 May 1984 issue of *Science* — almost exactly two years after his pledge that he would find the cause of AIDS within that time.

A press conference was called before publication, and in a bizarre outburst of fervent US nationalism, Gallo was hailed by senior American government officials as the virtual saviour of an embattled world. Secretary of Health and Human Services, Margaret Heckler, predicted that test kits for screening blood donations for the AIDS virus would be ready in six months and that a vaccine would be developed in two years. (By 1986, blood tests had indeed been introduced widely, but there was absolutely no sign of a vaccine. In fact, by 1986, the official target date for getting an AIDS vaccine ready for public use had been put back to the year 2000. Not for the first time a senior official who should have known better had made dangerous pronouncements for political and nationalistic reasons.)

By the time Gallo's results were published in 1984, the French had also made great improvements to their own AIDS test, which was based on antibodies to their LAV virus. The French were also showing that the presence of their virus was closely associated with symptoms of AIDS. Interestingly, their work was done with help from the CDC in Atlanta — an indication that co-operation in AIDS research between the two countries was still possible even at that relatively late stage. Indeed, shortly before publication of his research papers on HTLV-3, Gallo visited the Pasteur Institute to lecture on retroviruses. 'I came back to the United States happy, confident and feeling the best feelings I have had', Gallo later recalled. His good humour would not last long, however.

Certainly the fanfare which surrounded publication of Gallo's papers did nothing to help the already touchy Gallic chauvinism. This irritation quickly turned to fury when the French scientists read Gallo's papers for themselves. They found the their own pioneering work had been virtually ignored. Gallo merely noted that the French had isolated a retrovirus but rated their research as being too poorly developed to merit comment. An enraged Montagnier told reporters he was 'shocked' and pointed out his team had done important work in analysing the virus's structure, had shown that it infected T4 cells, and had gone a long way themselves in developing an antibody test that could be used to screen blood donors and people in high risk groups.

Gallo has proved to be equally sensitive, if not more so, on other occasions. During a visit to London's Imperial Cancer Research Fund headquarters, Gallo amazed researchers with his fury at the sight of copies of *New Scientist* in its library. The journal had carried an editorial sympathetic to some of Montagnier's claims, causing a furious Gallo to denounce it as a rag and to suggest the journals be thrown out!

But the real question remained unanswered. Which virus was the true cause of AIDS — LAV or HTLV-3? The answer was not long in coming — and when it did, there were some shocked reactions. Using powerful, modern biological analytic techniques, scientists found that LAV and HTLV-3 were simply variants of the same virus. The French were furious. They had identified the virus a full year before Gallo. Yet he had received all the glory while they been ignored. Gallo had quite deliberately stolen their credit, they maintained — and some of Gallo's fellow American scientists agreed. Never a popular figure because of his bombastic approach to his own research, Gallo was described by one unnamed American scientist, quoted in *Discover*, as being 'as opportunistic as a virus himself '.

In defence of Gallo and his team, other Americans pointed out that the French had still been unable to prove that their virus was the cause of AIDS and had not been able to study its structure properly. That was the real achievement of the team from the National Cancer Institutes, they said. The dispute sounded petty but the stakes were extremely high. Apart from the matter of prestige and awards, possibly even a Nobel prize, there are high financial rewards for those who can market a patented test for spotting carriers of a disease like AIDS. These rewards are reckoned to be for sums of several million dollars in the case of the AIDS test and have been the real cause of the rancour and bitter feuding between the French and the Americans.

The French view is not hard to understand. They were the first to isolate HTLV3/LAV — as most scientists now diplomatically label the virus — and they also filed the first patent for an antibody test based upon that discovery. (The Pasteur scientists filed in September 1983 in Europe and in December in the United States. Gallo, on the other hand, did not file his patent in the US until April 1984.) Despite the priority of the French patent claim, however, it was Gallo's application that was granted by the US government in 1985. A year after this pronouncement, the French were still waiting for a decision on their case.

Neither Gallo or Montagnier or their research teams stand to gain personally. The patents for the two tests are held by the US government and the Pasteur Institute — the employers of Gallo and Montagnier — and they are the real beneficiaries. Both stand to earn considerable sums by licensing out their systems to pharmaceutical companies who want to maufacture and sell AIDS antibody tests. Such tests will always be needed throughout the world, as medical authorities strive to halt the spread of AIDS. It is estimated that in America alone, the revenue from licensing antibody tests will be about $5 million a year by the end of the decade.

Without a US patent, the French could not market their own test in the US, which was to have been maufactured under licence by the drug company, Genetic Systems Corporation of Seattle. If they had marketed their test, the French would have had to pay royalties to the US government, the owner of the only patent granted in America for an AIDS antibody test. It was an infuriating prospect for an institute whose scientists considered themselves to be the original discoverers of the AIDS virus and were the first to apply for a patent. As a result, the French began to press for compensation.

A meeting was arranged between the Pasteur Institute's representatives and senior US government health officials — who discovered the French were seeking a lot more than just the granting of their outstanding patient application. They were also demanding that the US recognize the Pasteur Institute as the real discoverers of the AIDS virus; that the US patent be declared invalid; and that it only be reissued with the French named as co-holders.

In fact, the French were suggesting (although they did not openly say so) that the virus discovered by Gallo, and on which the US patent was based, was actually the one discovered by Montagnier. It was certainly true that samples of LAV had been sent to Gallo, at his request, just before his team's crucial breakthrough. However, Gallo says he could not get Montagnier's virus samples to grow in his laboratory. Nevertheless, the French stuck to their guns, and pointed out how remarkably similar are the two strains isolated by Gallo and Montagnier. (Scientists know that a single type of virus — for instance, the influenza virus — can vary a great deal in its structure and very different strains have been found in patients with the same symptoms. The HTLV-3 and LAV strains isolated by Montagnier and Gallo were unusually similar.)

The virus sent to Gallo was intended for research purposes only, said the French. Instead, they have implied that Gallo used it to develop his test — a procedure that would be in direct contravention of all agreed practices for controlling scientific co-operation between laboratories. It is an extremely serious allegation, amounting to an accusation that Gallo was guilty of scientific misconduct, says the journal *Science*. Not surprisingly Gallo angrily denies the allegation. The two viruses are not identical, he says. Anyway, he adds, Montagnier did not send him a big enough sample for him to carry out proper experiments.

Nevertheless, the French have persisted with their attack, while the US government has refused — with equal stubborness — to give ground. As a result, in December 1985, the French announced they would no longer negotiate and instead decided to sue the US government. It is a dispiriting finale to a remarkable scientific detective story, for in many ways both sides can take great credit for their endeavours. Within a mere three years of uncovering a dangerous new disease, the scientists pinpointed the offending virus and did much to characterize its structure and behaviour.

Gallo takes credit for first pinpointing retroviruses as the cause of AIDS, for laying the research groundwork, and — once he had finally isolated the virus — for firmly establishing that it was truly the cause of AIDS. For his part, Montagnier was the first to identify that HTLV-3/LAV was the guilty virus and to recognize its power to kill T-cells. His Pasteur Institute team was also the first to file a patent for a desperately needed AIDS antibody test. Many scientists consider it is a marvel that both achieved so much in such a brief period. Their work reflects the astonishing progress that has been made in molecular biology recently. Indeed, many believe that if AIDS had appeared ten years before it did, the chances of unravelling its secrets would have been dramatically reduced.

Sensitive US feelings were not helped by the decision of

the dying Rock Hudson to travel to France to seek treatment with drugs that were not available in the United States. His decision — tragically futile as it was — had the beneficial effect of galvanizing the US Congress for the first time. The failure of his last ditch battle cruelly underlined the fact that America was doing little to help the plight of an estimated 15,000 people who had by then contracted AIDS. Congress pledged a staggering $240 million for AIDS research and promised more for the near future. Politicians were vitually writing a blank cheque in their desperation to solve a problem that was assuming frightening proportions.

The French also reacted hastily, and sometimes with less beneficial effects. In October 1985, three doctors at Paris's Laennec Hospital — Philippe Even, Jean-Marie Andrieu and Alain Venet — announced they had made a dramatic breakthrough in slowing and countering the ravages of AIDS in victims already in advanced stages of the disease. This 'miracle cure' was named as cyclosporin-A.

It seemed a strange candidate for an anti-AIDS drug. Cyclosporin-A is normally used to slow down the immune system during transplant surgery in a bid to prevent the body rejecting an organ which it might otherwise consider to be 'foreign'. In AIDS victims, with already depleted immune systems, their conditions would surely be expected only to worsen, it seemed. But as Philippe Even, the team's leader, explained at the time: 'The AIDS virus can only move against active T-cells. We therefore had the idea of reducing that activity by giving them an immune suppressant, cyclosporin-A'.

The three doctors' 'triumph' was announced to the world at a press conference attended by France's health minister, Mrs Georgina Dufoix. The occasion had all the depressing memories of the announcement of Gallo's discoveries the previous year. There was certainly no shortage of national fervour. However, there did seem to be a distinct lack of hard scientific fact to go with it. When the team duly revealed that trials had only been carried out on two patients, enthusiasm for their 'breakthrough' began to wane. Within a fortnight, the remaining gloss was removed when one of their two 'recovering' test cases died. The French newspapers denounced the team for its premature disclosure of results and the scientists were accused of blatantly attempting to steal a march on American rivals. Indeed, Even subsequently admitted in the journal *Nature* that there had been strong government pressure on them to announce success of their drug before carrying out proper tests. 'It was not our decision — it was the minister of health's', he said, although he did not explain how the minister had first been informed of their work. The damage done to AIDS victims, whose hopes had been falsely raised by claims for cyclosporin-A was incalculable, however.

The bitterness of the battle between the Americans and the French has even extended to a struggle over the naming of the AIDS virus. Gallo is adamant that it should be labelled HTLV-3. Montagnier is equally sure that it should be called LAV. As a result, a committee has been set up to settle the issue.

The committee will also have to deliberate on a third, less well-known candidate, ARV, or AIDS-related virus, which was isolated independently by Jay Levy, of the University of California at San Francisco, and which has subsequently been shown to be the same virus as that discovered by Gallo and Montagnier.

Once again it seems that the two sides have locked themselves into a petty and rather irrelevant argument. But, in fact, there are other important issues at stake. The fundamental disagreement centres on a dispute over which family of viruses is really responsible for AIDS. On one side Gallo is sure that the AIDS virus is the third member of the Human T-cell Leukaemia Virus family that he first identified in 1978. The reasons are clear, he says. There are only three known human retroviruses and they all attack T-cells in the blood. In addition, there are significant similarities in genetic structure between all these three viruses. But

Montagnier disputes this. He and his Pasteur Institute team have come to the conclusion that the AIDS virus is really a form of lentivirus — a micro-organism of the same family as the visna virus which causes disease in sheep but which has never before been linked to human disease.

In making this claim, Montagnier points to the newest, and one of the most worrying aspects of the AIDS story. It is the discovery that the disease now appears to be producing frequent signs of brain damage. Indeed, in 10 per cent of cases, it is neurological damage that gives the first indication that the patient is suffering from AIDS. As further evidence, the French team also points out that the genetic structures of the AIDS virus and the lentivirus are very similar. At present there are only three known types of lentivirus — one which causes brain infections in sheep; another that produces infectious anaemia in horses, and a third that causes encephalitis in goats. Little else is known of these three variants — apart from the fact that on infecting domestic animals, the resulting infections are so pernicious and unresponsive to drugs that the creatures invariably have to be put down.

For this part, Gallo has changed his original stance, which he had outlined in his 1984 lectures on AIDS (he is, incidently, a gifted speaker). Then he argued that HTLV-1 and -3 are really variants of the same virus. In the case of HTLV-1, T-cells are transformed into malignant versions of themselves and spread through the body to cause a type of leukaemia. In the case of HTLV-3, the target is still the T-cells which are killed instead. The target is the same, the crucial T-cell mechanism of the immune system, only the method of attack is slightly different. Indeed, Gallo even speculated that the waves of HTLV-3 infections which have spread round the world causing AIDS would be followed by similar but slower-acting HTLV-1 infections which would cause parallel but delayed epidemics of leukaemia.

But later Gallo modified these assertions and actually acknowledged there were similarities between the AIDS virus and the lentivirus family and that there were fewer parallels with the HTLV family than he had first supposed.

The rest of the scientific world is divided. Some scientists even suggest that the AIDS virus is neither an HTLV or a lentivirus but is of a completely new type. Resolving the issue is of crucial importance, however. (Nor should it be thought that only French and US scientists have made all the important breakthroughs. For instance, British researchers at the Chester Beatty Institute in London were responsible for carrying out crucial research that showed that the virus attacked only cells that carried T4 receptor sites. This was a particularly important step in uncovering the virus's attack route.)

Much effort is going into the solution of this problem and already scientists have learned a great deal, not just about the AIDS virus and its impact, but about the techniques employed by our bodies to tackle invading micro-organisms.

This is one of the rare benefits of the AIDS tragedy. It has shed new light on the mysterious workings of our immune systems and also revealed much about the way viruses wreak damage. As Dr Dalgleish put it: 'AIDS has been a tragedy in human terms but it has also provided scientists with a new source of stimulation. AIDS has done for medical research what the Second World War did for the aircraft industry.'

* Gallo subsequently changed this nomenclature to Human T-Lymphotropic Virus.

5

Armies in Retreat

Like tiny armies, our bodies' immune systems are poised to protect us against all manner of aggression. Without their defensive power, we would be exposed to an uncountable range of attacks from invading micro-organisms and poisons. We would quickly sicken and die. Indeed, in many ways, the military analogy is a good one, for the immune system is organized on a sound soldierly command structure. It has three elements.

The first stage is called *induction* and is the equivalent of the operation of an army's spy or intelligence network. Enemy troops – the invading microbes – are spotted and the rest of the immune system is alerted, just as an army's HQ would be kept informed about the movements of its foe.

The second stage is known as *regulation*, and mirrors the actions that would take place at headquarters once the enemy has been observed and identified. A plan is prepared and orders are issued to implement it.

The final part of the operation is carried out by the *effectors,* the body's own troops, which swarm into battle to defend us. Some of the most frequently employed of these 'soldiers' are the antibodies, which are rapidly manufactured by parts of the immune system called the B-cells. The antibodies then rush to the battlefield, surround the enemy micro-organisms, block their chemical actions and prevent them from attacking or breaking into cells.

However, we have more than one type of 'soldier' at our disposal. Some of the most important of these other defenders are the macrophages, which can engulf and digest entire microbes. Other vital components of our immune defences include the granulocytes (or neutrophils) which also ingest organisms, and chemicals such as interferons.

And at the centre of all these complex activities, the T-cell plays a crucial role. The T-cell is manufactured in bone marrow and then migrates through our bodies in a partially developed form until it reaches the thymus, a gland at the base of the neck. The thymus then gives the immature T-cell a final set of chemical instructions which transforms it into one of three adult forms — a *killer,* a *helper,* or a *suppressor* T-cell. The killer T-cell defends the body by attacking invading cells by disrupting their cell membranes, a process called *lysing.* The suppressor T-cell has the job of shutting down the body's immune response once an infection has been dealt with. That leaves us with the T4, or T-helper, cell.

The influence of the T-helper is profound. The other T-cells cannot function without its controlling influence. In addition, it secretes chemicals, such as interleukin-2 and gamma-interferon which stimulate other parts of the immune system so they are properly prepared to defend an attack. In this way T-helpers are responsible for 'arming', or preparing, macrophages so they can engulf and destroy invaders. If macrophages are not armed, some enemy organisms can survive inside them and may possibly breed and grow.

The T-helper also plays a vital role in the production of antibodies, the 'foot soldiers' of our immune systems. The B-cells, which act as production lines for manufacturing antibodies, require a signal from T-helpers before they can begin their work. The T-helper is clearly a vital component of our anti-disease defences and is normally well protected at the heart of the immune system. Only an extremely evasive organism could successfully overcome it — a description that fits the AIDS virus exactly.

Indeed, the virus possesses a staggering array of weapons. For one thing, the AIDS virus can delude the body's defences into manufacturing the wrong sorts of antibodies. Instead of manufacturing antibodies that will latch onto crucial, active parts of the virus, the immune system makes antibodies that attach themselves to unimportant parts of the virus, leaving it free to attack cells. In addition, the AIDS virus can also change the chemical make-up of its coat so that it becomes even harder to identify and attack. More important, by making a first strike at the very heart of our disease defences it can deal them a mortal blow. As Jeffrey Laurence, assistant professor of medicine at the Cornell University Medical Center in New York, states: 'The AIDS virus has little need for evasion for it avoids destruction by pre-emptively destroying the immune system'.

It is certainly a well-armed virus. As Gallo states:

One way a virus can escape the immune system is to directly attack it. The AIDS virus does that. Another way a virus can escape the immune system is to change its coat. The AIDS virus does that. A virus can also get round the body's defences by putting a lot of sugars round its own coat so that antibodies will not attack the virus so well. This virus does that more than any other retrovirus we have seen. And in addition, a virus can try to avoid detection by hiding and not being expressed until certain moments. The AIDS virus does that as well.

The virus first attacks by attaching one section of itself to a particular molecule on the surface of a T-helper cell. The virus sections fits into the cell molecule like a key fits into a lock and opens up the cell membrane, allowing the virus to get inside the T-helper. Once inside, the virus first sheds its protective chemical coat, exposing its core which is made of the genetic material RNA. Then it uses the enzyme reverse transcriptase to make a DNA copy of itself. This copy is then inserted into the cell's own DNA. Once that has happened the integrated virus cannot be distinguished from the rest of the genes inside the cell.

In this state, the virus can lie dormant for months, possibly years, before it becomes activated and begins to spread. Scientists say this probably occurs when the T-helper cell itself begins to replicate in response to an infection by another virus or bacteria. When the cell's reproductive machinery is switched on, it starts making more copies of the virus as well. This is a normal process with other viruses once they become lodged inside an infected cell's DNA. But the AIDS virus has an extra trick up its sleeve. It possesses a key chemical component which enables it to have its own genes read out far more efficiently and quickly than the cell's own DNA. This component is called TAT (transacting transcriptional regulation) and it allows the growth of the virus to speed up enormously.

After a while, viral 'buds' begin to appear on the outside of the T-helper cell and these break off to move on to infect more cells, completing the life-cycle of the AIDS virus. The original T-helper is eventually killed in the process. Once a critical number of cells have been destroyed in this way, the depletion of the immune system cannot be reversed. A devastating chain of events, triggered by the loss of T-cells, is set in motion. As Jeffrey Laurence describes in *Scientific American:* 'Lacking T-helper cell help, B-cells are unable to produce enough antibodies to the AIDS virus or to any other infection. The killer T-cell response is similarly hampered. Suppressor T-cells cannot fulfil their role either.' The immune system is crippled and the body can no longer fight off microbial attack.

Dealing with a virus that attacks in such a pernicious way poses enormous problems for those scientists trying to develop cures and treatments for AIDS. Only medicines that can kill every infected cell and mop up all the free viruses in the blood will be able to deal with the virus. Its ability to lie in a dormant state for longer periods also poses problems. Without manifest symptoms, victims — and carriers — can infect others without realizing they are passing on infection.

This dangerous power has an unusual source. Retro-viruses are in fact very poor at reproducing once inside the body. For one thing, they are slow reproducers, which explains why they lie in a quiescent, but still dangerous, state for such long periods. In addition, the AIDS virus also replicates rather inefficiently — mistakes frequently appear in the copies that spread from infected T-helper cells. This may be how the virus changes its structure. It is simply a by-product of its poor reproductive ability.

Fortunately, the AIDS virus is made less dangerous because it is reasonably difficult to pass on. Transmission needs direct insertion into the bloodstream from contaminated syringes, blood, or genital secretions. Doctors believe that infected blood that falls on skin or food does not pose a hazard.

In the first AIDS cases discovered in America, scientists believe the main transmission route was from semen to blood. Those infected were usually highly promiscuous gays and among them doctors found that the act of receptive anal sex appeared to carry a particularly high risk. This has been confirmed in other studies which have shown that the passive partner in relationships is the one in special danger. This is explained by scientists who speculate that the wall of the rectum is extremely fragile and is likely to be easily ruptured and broken during anal sex. Semen infected with the AIDS virus, or possibly carrying infected T-cells (which are known to be present in semen) can then pass into the passive partner's blood stream. However, active partners have also contracted AIDS. The tissue at the tip of the penis is very fragile, and is also prone to tearing during disruptive sexual acts, so the blood of both partners can mingle, passing on the AIDS virus to the active partner.

With heterosexual couples the transmission may be more difficult. The vagina is certainly a much hardier place than the rectum, its lining walls being far less prone to penetration by micro-organisms. Others believe that emphasis on differences between hetero- and homosexual routes will give a false and dangerous sense of security. They point to cases of artificially inseminated women in Australia who were infected, suggesting that it is not that hard to transmit among heterosexuals. Indeed, there has been a steady increase in the number of cases in which the disease has spread between heterosexuals. In Africa, victims are often promiscuous men and women, and doctors there have reported that AIDS is particularly associated with people with histories of other sexually transmitted diseases such as syphilis or herpes. Some scientists speculate that the effects of these diseases may be involved in easing the spread of the AIDS virus. The sores and wounds which are the symptoms of such venereal diseases will greatly increase the chances of an exchange and mingling of blood, producing infections, they say.

Other doctors do not believe such explanations are necessary. The simple passage of the virus from semen to the vagina may be enough to pass on the disease. And if homosexual active partners can pick up the virus through their penile tissue during anal intercourse, then so too could heterosexual men during vaginal intercourse, it is argued. A problem still remains in attempting to explain how the vagina becomes infected, as its walls are tougher. One study, greeted with great interest at the 'AIDS in Africa' conference in November 1985, suggested an explanation. In this study, carried out at the pathobiology and urology department at Wisconsin University in the US, the investigators found that in some parts of a woman's cervix populations of T-helper cells are found to survive. They may then be involved in transmission of the AIDS virus.

Parents can pass on AIDS to their offspring. When this occurs, the prognosis for the infected child is particularly poor, as the infant's immature immune system is probably even less capable of resisting the virus than an adult's. By April 1985, in the US there had been 113 cases of children who had contracted AIDS. Among victims there were just as many girls as boys and most had one or both parents in a high AIDS risk group. Scientists are still unsure about the main route of transmission in such cases. They believe that the disease is either passed from mother to offspring when the virus diffuses through the placenta during pregnancy or that it is passed on in mother's milk after birth. The former explanation is considered much more probable, though the latter can occur. In Sydney, Australia, in July 1985, a case in which the virus was passed to a child after being breast fed was recorded. It is thought that the mother was infected during a blood transfusion that was carried out after she had given birth.

There is a possibility that fathers can also pass on AIDS to their children. Male haemophiliacs have certainly given the disease to their offspring — though this is thought to occur because mothers have been infected during normal sexual intercourse. They have then passed on the virus to the offspring they were carrying.

The AIDS virus has also been found in the saliva of some victims — a discovery that has raised the possibility that the virus could be passed on by kissing or in water droplets expelled during coughing or sneezing. However, careful study of cases has revealed absolutely no supporting evidence — although Gallo has said he does believe that HTLV3/LAV may be transmitted during very heavy exchanges of saliva. Most other doctors believe that sex and blood transfers are by far the most important routes for the transmission of AIDS.

Once the virus has been passed on, there can be a considerable delay in the onset of symptoms. Indeed, when the first cases were reported it was thought there this latency period could last for many years. Recent research has slightly altered this picture, however. In cases where AIDS has been passed on through infected blood products, doctors have been able to trace and pinpoint the exact time of first infection. Similarly, by carefully questionning infected gays and drug users and by then tracing partners, it has been possible to nail down exact times of infections in some cases. Now doctors believe that the average latency period of the disease is 28 months although it can vary between six months and six years — the limit of our observations so far.

When symptoms do appear, they often arrive in the form

of swollen lymph glands. These glands are a crucial part of the body's defence systems. They are linked together as part of the lymph system and each gland acts as a munitions factory for the immune system. They often swell when we are suffering from viral or bacterial infections as they begin to gear up for action with killer T-cells and antibodies spilling off production lines and departing for war. But in cases of HTLV3/LAV infection, the swelling is a direct result of infection and is not a by-product of the body's responses to other infections. In other illnesses, the enlargement of the glands — which lie behind the ears, round the collar bone, at the elbows, in the groin, behind the knee, under the arms and in other sites — passes away after a few days or weeks. This does not happen with HTLV3/LAV infections. The glands remain enlarged and a person is described as suffering from *PGL* — persistent generalized lymphadenopathy. PGL is a less severe form of infection, and in most cases it does not lead to AIDS. Not all HTLV3/LAV infected people suffer from PGL, nor does the presence of PGL mean a person is going to succumb to AIDS itself. Many appear to survive initial infection with HTLV3/LAV.

There are other signs that reveal the presence of HTLV3/LAV, however. The patient can suffer from one or all of the following — unexplained exhaustion, bouts of fever, intense attacks of sweating during sleep, weight loss of up to 10 lb (4.5 kg), and diarrhoea. These may be the effects of early opportunistic infections. For instance cytomegalovirus (which is commonly associated with AIDS) often causes fevers. All these symptoms are fairly innocuous and are quite common in other minor illnesses. This can be disturbing for people who believe that they are at risk of getting AIDS or fear that they may have become infected. The occurence of everyday complaints — such as headaches or indigestion — can all too easily be interpreted as the first signs of AIDS, and a daily ritual of frantic symptom-hunting can be set in motion.

Doctors have found that less obvious, but more indicative changes take place during infection. Normally a healthy individual has about five T-helper cells to every two or three T-suppressor cells in their blood. In some AIDS cases this ratio can be reversed, revealing that serious depletion of T-helper cells has occurred — a clear sign that the immune system itself is under deadly attack.

In cases of full-blown Acquired Immune Deficiency Syndrome, severe opportunistic infections develop. They include: fungal infections that cause candida growths (thrush) in the mouth, throat and oesophagus; protozoal infections that cause PCP pneumonia or toxoplasmosis; viruses like herpes simplex which produce genital lesions and eye infections; and bacteria which cause salmonella, blood poisoning and tuberculosis. Other opportunistic infections include viruses and fungi that attack the brain producing lethargy, chronic depression and dementia. These operate in addition to the HTLV3/LAV's own attacks on the central nervous system.

About 40 per cent of AIDS patients are now thought to suffer severe neurological damage. Much of this is directly produced by HTLV3/LAV which is revealing itself in a new role — as a primary cause of cell damage. For instance, in cases where no opportunistic infections have been observed causing brain tumours, it has still been found that victims can no longer function at their work, undergo personality alterations, exhibit a marked atrophy of their grey matter, and suffer grand mal epilepsy in addition to dementia, report scientists writing in *The Management of AIDS Patients* (Miller, D. *et al.*, 1986, Macmillan Press). Similarly, James Holland and Richard Price, at New York's Memorial Sloan-Kettering Cancer Center have found that many of their AIDS patients developed a severe form of dementia that caused slurred speech, slow movements, loss of memory and psychosis.

Others have found evidence of specific psychiatric disorders that are quite separate from the psychological conditions that develop as reactions to AIDS and the prospects of death. For instance, one group of University of California in Los Angeles scientists found 'clinically impressive' evidence that language disorders can occur. Victims reveal 'marked limitations in the complexity of their sentence structures and show very slow verbal responses', report the psychiatrists, Drs Wolcott, Fawzy and Pasnau. 'These language disorders have been found in patients with no other evidence of dementia. The symptoms may fluctuate from day to day and are sometimes associated with movement disorders'.

Some scientists believe that the AIDS virus infects the brain because many neurological cells have chemcial markers on them that are similar to those on the outside of T-cells. They therefore become targets for the virus as well. Others suggest that brain cells may become infected when diseased T-cells fuse with them. Either way the evidence — that HTLV3/LAV appears to produce clinical symptoms of its own — changes many previous assumptions about AIDS. As a result, scientists, including Gallo, now believe that the very name 'Acquired Immune Deficiency Syndrome' no longer adequately sums up the variety of different conditions produced by the virus and that a completely new, all-encompassing title should be found.

The discovery of HTLV3/LAV brain damage has also prompted some doctors to make fairly apocalyptic forecasts about future death rates among carriers. At present the standard death rate from infection is quoted as being about 10 per cent. This figure is based upon studies of blood samples taken from a few groups of American gays in 1980 during studies of other diseases. Following the outbreak of AIDS, doctors went back to these samples and found many had been HTLV3/LAV carriers at the time. Since then an estimated figure of 'at least 10 per cent' have contracted full-blown AIDS and are not expected to recover.

Privately, many senior scientists admit that they consider this figure to be an absolute minimum. For instance, one scientist involved in such studies, Dr Donald Francis, of California's Health and Welfare Agency in Berkeley has found that among some of these early HTLV3/LAV carriers, fatalities have risen to about 25 per cent. 'At least 10 per cent will definitely develop AIDS' he says. 'The evidence suggests that that proportion will be higher and that other AIDS related conditions, including encephalopathic conditions, will occur at increasing rates with time'. This view is backed by Professor Robin Weiss, of London's Institute of Cancer Research who takes a 'rather pessimistic view'. He says that 'quite a high proportion of infected people some time or other will develop severe disease.'

Other doctors have been even more alarmist — such as Drs Cecil and Cottler Fox, whose letter on AIDS and the human brain was published by *Nature* in 1986. Basing their argument on the interpretation that the AIDS virus is 'akin to the lentiviruses' as Montagnier suggests, they estimate that between 100,000 and 1,000,000 Americans may develop serious brain disease as a result of HTLV3/LAV infection by the end of the century. 'The implications of such a large number of men, women and children with progressive disease for the economy, health care system and emotional state of society are unprecedented', they claim.

In a special editorial written in response to the letter, the editor of *Nature,* John Maddox says that the communication is 'plainly written to scare but should be taken seriously for all that'. He adds:

It is reasonable to expect that in due course the infection will spread through the general population in the narrow sense that the groups now most at risk will be less conspicuous. That is what seems to have happened in some parts of central Africa.
 Articles in the clinical journals also point to a neurological component of AIDS. More ominously, some of those in whose nervous tissue HTLV3/LAV has been found are people without overt AIDS. What would happen if psychiatric hospitals were filled with relatively young people suffering from conditions at

present associated with old age, dementia for example? Could we shoulder the burden? The question is chilling.

But brain cells and T-cells cannot be the only victims of the AIDS virus, say scientists. It is becoming clear that HTLV3/LAV also attacks other cells in the body.

Says Dr Pinching:

I don't think that the loss of T-helper cells can be the sole cause of the destruction of immune systems. Our immune defences are very sophisticated and highly complex and have many failsafe mechanisms.

You can appreciate that when you look at children who suffer from natural immune deficiencies. If only one part of their immune system is knocked out before birth, they do not have too much trouble surviving. Other parts of the system take over from the missing section. There have to be two or more parts of the system knocked out before the consequences become really severe.

That is why I think that, within the immune system, the AIDS virus infects more than just the T-cell. Macrophages and other related cells are also infected. That would explain the severity of the impact of AIDS on the immune system.

Certainly, the action of the AIDS virus is now being appreciated as being one of great complexity and appears to go beyond the fairly straightforward picture that was once painted of it wiping out the immune system at a stroke. As Jeffrey Laurence states in *Scientific American*: 'A decrease in the number of T-helper cells cannot account for the full extent of the immune defects seen in AIDS patients. In the early stages of the disease, for example, patients may still have a normal number of T-helper cells and yet their immune defenses are already severely weakened.' This statement is supported by the observations of other scientists who have found that the symptoms of the disease — the brain disorders, the opportunistic infections and tumours — can occur without any sign of damage to T-cells. One suggestion is that the virus somehow triggers the body's immune system so that it attacks its own T-helper cells. The antibodies created to do this may attack not just infected T-helpers but also block the action of uninfected T-helpers, severely impairing the efficiency of the immune system.

But the strange behaviour of the AIDS virus and the T-helpers is not the only puzzle about the disease. The most basic of these is summed up by the simple question: Why do some opportunist infections affect AIDS victims while others do not? It is indeed a fascinating problem. If the immune system is so severely compromised in AIDS why is the list of associated infections relatively limited? As Dr Pinching says: 'This disease is telling us something extremely important about the body but we cannot unscramble the exact message as yet'. As AIDS has only appeared on the scene relatively recently, scientists have had relatively little chance to decode the message. Nevertheless, many are confident they will learn a great deal from studying AIDS.

One of the most intriguing problems about AIDS is the prevalance among victims of the cancer Kaposi's sarcoma (named after the Austrian dermatologist Dr Moritz Kohn Kaposi who first identified it in 1872). Symptoms of the disease first appear in the form of purple or blue patches on the skin of the lower body, especially the feet. In time both feet and hands become deformed from the thickening of affected areas of skin. Lesions form and also affect the scalp, mouth, throat, stomach and intestines. Nodules appear, disappear and return, some eventually turning ulcerous. Many patients report burning or itching feelings in their hands and feet. The sarcoma is unusual among cancers because it appears to originate in several areas of the body at the same time. Most other cancers are thought to arise at a single site when a cell becomes malignant. Kaposi's sarcoma was extremely rare in America and Europe before 1980. Mainly affecting elderly men of Jewish or Mediterranean origin, less than one case per million of the population was reported in the US. With the spread of AIDS, Kaposi's prevalence has shot up. But why has this extremely rare cancer attacked AIDS victims in particular while other cancers have not? It is extremely puzzling.

But perhaps more intriguing is the difference in prevalence rates of the sarcoma (the word comes from the Greek for 'fleshy growth') among different groups of AIDS patients. In homosexual patients with AIDS the risk of contracting Kaposi's is about five times that of patients from any of the other risk groups. In all about 44 per cent of all homosexual AIDS victims develop the tumour. It is not at all clear why that should be. However, many scientists now speculate that a second virus may be responsible for causing Kaposi's sarcoma — one that may particularly affect homosexuals. This insight into the possible involvement of a new virus that is associated with cancer in humans is one of the most exciting features of the story of AIDS.

Another puzzling aspect to the disease is that in small numbers of cases infected people do not produce detectable antibodies. Patients can begin to display symptoms of the disease but when tested produce negative results. However, using far more laborious techniques, scientists are able to sample their blood and can directly detect the presence of HTLV3/LAV in their cells (rather than the virus's antibody). It is a worrying discovery. The development of the HTLV3/LAV test — which relies on the detection of antibodies — is still the best way to prevent infected carriers donating blood or passing on the virus in other ways. The recognition that it is not infallible means that people in high risk groups must still *not* donate blood.

But probably the most intriguing question is this: Where on Earth did AIDS come from? An answer to that would be particularly valuable in developing treatments and cures. Many scientists are sure they now know the answer — that AIDS originated in Africa. It is an assertion that has provoked a great deal of anger and controversy.

6

Out of Africa

At first glance, the setting for the first international symposium on 'AIDS in Africa' was ideal. The elegant and well-appointed Brussels Congress Centre is a perfect venue for any international scientific meeting. And gathered at the Brussels conference were many of the most respected names in AIDS research — Gallo, Montagnier, Clumeck, Weiss, Francis, Tedder, and others. It was surely the perfect opportunity for discussing one of the most urgent and alarming aspects of AIDS — its rapid spread through men and women in central Africa.

Only on second glance did it become clear that one, vital, ingredient was missing. There were hardly any Africans at the symposium. Of the 600 delegates, only a few dozen Africans could be seen in a sea of Western scientists and journalists. It was a puzzling and disturbing sight. For the previous two years, AIDS had been spreading dramatically among young heterosexuals in cities such as Kigali and Nairobi. Why should central African states shrug aside a chance to learn about this tragic new scourge? And why should they refuse to co-operate with Western scientists in discussing the horrifying worldwide implications of the African AIDS epidemic? Delegates soon found out.

From the beginning of the symposium, the few African delegates who did attend made their feelings clear. They accused Americans and Europeans of spreading alarmist and inaccurate stories on the prevalence of AIDS in African cities. They claimed these reports would seriously jeopardize their countries' tourist industries, a vital source of foreign currency.

In the months that preceded the Brussels symposium,

African politicians had already voiced similar feelings. Jeremiah Nyagah, Kenya's Minister for Environment and Natural Resources had denounced a European 'media campaign' which he said greatly exaggerated the extent of AIDS in his country. His outrage was particularly focused on a Swedish television programme which had claimed that 10 per cent of Kenya's population were carrying the AIDS virus. Mr Nyagah said these allegations were untrue and had been perpetrated as part of a 'smear campaign' against his country.

And in the week preceding the Brussels conference, Simon Shimeti, Kenya's permanent secretary at the Ministry of Health, had furiously rejected a *Boston Globe* story which suggested that AIDS was rampant in Central and East Africa. 'Just three people have died in this country — all of them expatriates. You can't call that rampant', he said. Significantly, he added: 'There is an element of racism in all this. AIDS surfaced in the United States but now they are saying that we are really to blame'. It was a view echoed by the African delegates at the Brussels conference. They were angered by Western researchers' repeated claims that Africa is the original source of the AIDS virus. They considered such an assertion to be an unjustified slur which had racist implications.

'How can they say that AIDS began in Africa?' asked Dr Chris Williams, a haematologist at Ibadan University, Nigeria, 'AIDS did not appear in Africa until after the disease had begun to spread in the United States. So how can they possibly suggest that we are responsible for AIDS?'

Many governments — including Kenya's — feared there would be so much hysterical publicity about AIDS in their countries that they put pressure on their own scientists and on foreign researchers working within their borders. Many invited delegates simply did not attend. Others suddenly and mysteriously cancelled at the last minute. It was a development which alarmed many scientists, particularly opening session chairman Professor Robin Weiss. He directly rebuked governments. 'If they are concerned about the public health of their people, and of people from elsewhere in the world, they cannot pretend that AIDS does not exist. Any individuals or countries who hope that by ignoring AIDS it will go away will be putting their people at hostage to suffering.'

Scientists have in fact shown considerable sympathy for African feelings. Nevertheless, they believe their research has clearly identified a massive epidemic of AIDS in Africa and that there is a link between the disease's early outbreak in the West and cases in rural central Africa. They see no slur in this observation. As Professor Jan Desmyter, of the Catholic University of Louvain in Belgium, put it: 'I have never heard of any stigma being attached to China, even though it is believed to be the origin of the influenza virus which has killed more people than AIDS'.

But the stigma of being the continent where AIDS originated is likely to stick. The insidious nature of AIDS itself and its associations with homosexual practices (considered to be taboo in many parts of Africa) has given the disease an unacceptable image. Scientists were warned to tread carefully. 'You must be extremely delicate in how you proceed if you are to avoid reviving the demons of racialism', warned the rector of the University of Brussels, M.H. Hasquin, during his speech to officially open the conference. 'Information on the spread of AIDS and Africa's involvement must be treated in a very careful, unemotional way.'

Getting hold of that information in a careful, unemotional way has not been so easy, however. Scientists carrying out AIDS research in central Africa have often had to work in extremely trying conditions. Many have been threatened with deportation after making 'unwise' statements to the Press, while others have been told to submit their research results for government clearance before sending them for publication in international journals. It is not the best climate in which to try to investigate a new and deadly epidemic.

In Zaire, where the first African AIDS cases were

reported, the government effectively banned all publicity about the disease. Scientists working there can only pass on their findings when they travel abroad. Other African countries have refused visas to journalists inquiring about AIDS. Even newspapers themselves have fallen foul of governments. The 9 November 1985, issue of the *International Herald Tribune* was banned outright by the Kenyan government because it contained an article which mentioned the existence of AIDS in the country. Similar pressures have been put on doctors and scientists from Africa itself. Lawrence Altman, a physician and also correspondent in Africa for the *New York Times* Service, recalls one African doctor who showed him two thick packs of green hospital record charts, one for AIDS cases, the other for suspected cases. 'These are growing thicker each week', he told Altman. 'Yet the director of the hospital tells me to tell officials that I have diagnosed only two cases of AIDS.'

Nevertheless, a fairly clear picture has emerged — and it has proved to be one of the most shocking and dramatic aspects of the AIDS story. Doctors have found evidence that a huge belt of Africa, stretching from Zaire to Rwandi, Burundi, Uganda, Tanzania, Kenya, and Zambia, is afflicted with an astonishingly high incidence of AIDS. The statistics quite dwarf European and American figures. In the cities of Zaire, for instance, it thought that one in ten people carry the AIDS virus. In Kinshasa, the capital, it was reported that there were 2,000 cases of AIDS in city hospitals by the beginning of 1985, and that this figure was rising. In another study, in Uganda, it was revealed that 20 per cent of tested citizens were found to be carriers. In every study, men and women were affected in roughly equal numbers, strongly suggesting that heterosexual contact is spreading the AIDS virus in Africa.

A striking example of this transmission — first from woman to man, and then from man to woman — was provided by Dr Clumeck. The case involved a wealthy

46-year-old Zairean man who died of AIDS in 1982. He had contracted the disease from a Zairean female prostitute, who also died of the disease. Before his death the Zairean man passed on the disease to four other women. All subsequently died of AIDS.

'From these cases, it is clear that normal sexual contact is involved in the transmission of AIDS', says Dr Clumeck. He points out that many female AIDS patients in both Zaire and Rwanda have been prostitutes or have had promiscuous husbands. One study of 33 Rwandan prostitutes revealed that 80 per cent had full-blown AIDS or related conditions. But even among the rest of the population of the tiny land-locked country of Rwanda, the incidence of the disease is staggering. It is thought that about one in twenty carry the virus and that by the end of the decade, about 25,000 Rwandans will have contracted AIDS.

Such a terrible toll in such a tiny country has enormous implications for the nation's meagre health resources. Already patients at the only hospital in Kigali, the capital, sometimes have to sleep two in a bed. Their families sleep outdoors in the hospital grounds and are required to feed their sick relative as the hospital lacks the cash to serve meals. Similar problems have been reported from other central African countries, such as Uganda. Dr Robert Downing, a virologist at Britain's Porton Down laboratories, recalls that the disease had reached 'devastating levels' when he co-operated with the slim disease research project described in Chapter 1.

'I came across one mission hospital where thirty of its 120 beds were occupied by AIDS victims. The disease has become a major health problem.'

In another study, of a group of Nairobi prostitutes, a team of Belgian and Kenyan scientists found that 64 per cent were carrying the AIDS virus and that one in three prostitutes working at a large hotel patronized by European tourists had AIDS antibodies in their blood. Crucially, other studies also revealed that the virus was spreading to prostitutes' customers. In 1980, 7 per cent of blood from one group of Kenyan prostitutes was found to contain antibodies to the AIDS virus; by 1984, it had reached 51 per cent. When their male customers were tested it was found that in 1980, 1 per cent were carrying the virus. In 1984, the percentage had increased to 13 per cent. A delayed, but parallel rise in virus-carrying men is occurring. And, as in the West, at least 10 per cent of all the infected people in these different studies will probably succumb to the full syndrome.

The problem has become so pervasive that a note of hysteria is creeping in. One columnist in a mass circulation Kenyan daily newspaper claimed that affected foreign tourists were purposely travelling to Africa in order to spread AIDS as part of a global conspiracy masterminded by multi-national drug companies who wanted 'to produce some Third World guinea-pigs'. Other ideas have a quainter ring. One Zairean prostitute told reporters that women got the disease from sleeping with dogs. Others claim AIDS is a white man's disease and say they have cut their contacts with Europeans and Americans to protect themselves.

Other countries affected by AIDS include Tanzania where cases have been found in western areas near Lake Victoria. The country's director of Preventive Medical Services, Dr Amani Meeni, publicly attributed the outbreak to the rise in prostitution in the area. This was 'the main factor in spreading AIDS', he said.

For such a new disease to become so well established in so many countries is a frightening development, and by 1985 signs were emerging that AIDS had also begun to move on to other parts of Africa. At the AIDS in Africa conference, Dr Williams of Ibadan University reported that a random sample of blood donors in Nigeria in West Africa had revealed that 7 per cent were carrying the AIDS virus. Other evidence of the disease's inexorable drift, this time to the south of Africa, was provided by Dr Ruben Sher, a pathologist from Johannesberg. He found a high incidence of the AIDS virus in the blood of men and women in a mining town in Zambia, in a random sample of men attending a sexual disease clinic in Malawi and among a small group of black workers in South Africa.

In all these cases, the virus responsible is HTLV3/LAV, the same one that has affected the West. And in all the studies it was found that men and women are affected in equal numbers. The implications for the rest of the world are extremely frightening.

However, there are aspects of AIDS in Africa that differ greatly from the disease in Europe and the US. A particularly striking difference is the number of children infected with the virus. 'Since nearly half the cases of AIDS in Africa occur among women in their reproductive years, and since these women are having many babies perinatal transmission is a very important problem', says Dr Peter Piot, a professor of microbiology at the Institute of Tropical Medicine at Antwerp, in Belgium, who has been closely involved in researching AIDS in Africa. The scale of the problem is revealed in the statistics on cases of AIDS in Rwanda. Of the 317 officially documented cases that had been reported by 1985, seventy of them (22 per cent) were children. This contrasts with figures from the US where less than 2 per cent of AIDS cases are infants.

Such figures are extremely depressing. Yet they probably disguise the true extent of the tragedy. Official health figures are notoriously unreliable in many African countries; countless other diseases and ailments — malaria, malnutrition, and others — can prevent doctors from recognizing the symptoms of AIDS; while victims often refuse to attend centres because they prefer the attentions of their native healers. All these factors conspire to conceal the seriousness of the problem. The rest of the world may have even less time than it thinks.

AIDS has rapidly taken a grip of Africa. But how could it do so in such an extraordinarily short time? Scientists have been baffled. 'Quite frankly, we don't know what is

happening', said Dr Fakhry Assaad, director of communi-
cable disease for the World Health Organization. 'There
must be special factors responsible for the spread of AIDS in
Africa but we just don't know what they are.' The search
for special African factors that would account for the
disease's particular course in the continent has been one of
the most absorbing parts of the AIDS story. After all, if AIDS
has spread so rapidly among African heterosexuals, it can
surely do the same in the West, unless unique African
factors are affecting the picture.

Scientists have offered a variety of suggestions. They
have proposed that AIDS may be spread by poor medical
practice, by anal intercourse which is used as a form of
contraception, or by biting insects. Certainly, efficient
medical practice is difficult to ensure in Africa, an
observation that supports the first theory. The costs of
disposable needles and a less than ideal attitude towards
proper medical cleanliness often mean that doctors and
health workers re-use syringes without properly sterilizing
them. The involvement of poor sterilization is backed by
African doctors themselves. Indeed, Dr Casimir Bizimungu,
director of the University Hospital, Butare, puts the blame
squarely on his own profession and accuses many of his
colleagues of using badly sterilized needles which
frequently pass on infection during vaccination programmes, and also during blood donations and
transfusions. 'The transmission of AIDS through sexual
relationships is rather rare', he says.

But if contaminated vaccines and transfusions are to
blame, there would be a general spread of AIDS cases
among all categories of people in the populations of central
Africa. But there is no sign of this. Cases are predominantly
made up of young, sexually active adults and their new-
born offspring.

The other 'special factor' theories also suffer from lack of
supporting evidence. One study of Rwandan prostitutes,
which showed that 88 per cent were carrying HTLV3/LAV,

found little evidence that they had practised anal intercourse. The researchers concluded that frequency of intercourse with different partners was more important than type of intercourse. As to the theory that mosquitos or other biting insects may be involved, this suffers from the same flaw as the contaminated needle proposal of Dr Bizimungu. Victims of all ages would be expected to go down with the disease. This is not the case.

From the beginning of the AIDS crisis in Africa, numbers of victims have been divided almost equally between men and women. The implications for the future course of the Western epidemic of AIDS are horrifying. Overall, most scientists now accept that heterosexual transmission is the main route of AIDS spread in Africa. In his book, *AIDS — The Acquired Immune Deficiency Syndrome* (MTP Press, 1985), Dr Victor Daniels states that evidence for such a route is now 'compelling'. And he adds that this 'could have disastrous consequences' for the rest of the world. However, he stresses that heterosexual transmission is not 'the complete answer' and that co-factors — such as the presence of other sexually transmitted diseases and infectious tropical diseases — may be involved in assisting the infectivity of the AIDS virus in Africa.

This view is backed by Dr Pinching. 'I certainly think AIDS is spread through normal heterosexual contacts, though we should be careful about how we interpret data from Africa. Certainly AIDS is undoubtedly going to be a world problem for both homosexuals and heterosexuals alike. Africa is telling us that people who think they are protected against AIDS because they are not homosexual are making a serious mistake.'

Equally, Dr Pinching rejects the idea put forward by some scientists who have suggested that European gays and African heterosexuals share a common susceptibility because of their lifestyles. Promiscuity or malnutrition might leave them immunologically deficient and open to infection from AIDS, it has been argued. 'There is little scientific validity in such ideas', says Dr Pinching. 'It is purely a matter of numbers of sexual contacts. The more you have the more you are likely to get AIDS'.

However, one co-factor that has probably assisted the spread of AIDS among young promiscuous men and women is the social upheaval now gripping much of Africa. There have been huge population shifts from rural communities to the cities of central Africa. These have not only thrown together large numbers of people and increased chances of sexual contact, but have also served to breakdown rigid social and tribal barriers that once would have acted as brakes on highly promiscuous living.

This is summed up by Alistair Matheson, *The Observer*'s correspondent in Nairobi: 'The traditionally conservative and closely knit family system seems to have suffered a traumatic breakdown in the face of sweeping urbanization in central Africa'. Matheson continues, 'Heterosexual promiscuity is now rampant in mushrooming towns and cities, and ethnic groups who have previously experienced very little contact with each other have been pitched almost overnight into a sexual melting pot. Researchers believe that it is in these rapidly changing circumstances that the AIDS virus has been able to spread at such an alarming pace.'

But there are other differences that separate AIDS in Africa from the disease that appears in the West. Apart from the obvious, crucial observation that there are different high risk groups — promiscuous heterosexuals in Africa and homosexuals in America and Europe — there is another intriguing divergence. Scientists have found the range of opportunistic infections afflicting victims is different from the range in the US and Europe.

One major example is the prevalence of PCP, the pneumocystis carinii pneumonia that has proved to be such a striking indicator of infection with HTLV3/LAV in the US. In Africa it is much less common, but skin diseases, cryptococcal meningitis, and a variety of intestinal complications appear more frequently. Such differences probably reflect the special types of viruses, fungi and other microbes that are common in Africa.

But there is another, more fundamental, puzzle thrown up by AIDS' particular manifestations in Africa; the discovery of a strange new type of Kaposi's sarcoma among victims. Before the appearance of AIDS, it was well established that Kaposi's sarcoma was endemic among African men. The cancer is about 200 times more prevalent there than in the US. There is even a special form of it that affects children. With the appearance of the first cases of AIDS, many doctors and scientists began to speculate — quite reasonably — that this history suggested AIDS could be an old African disease. HTLV3/LAV could have existed in Africa for centuries undetected among the many other ravaging illnesses there. Its presence would then explain the unusually high occurence of Kaposi's sarcoma there. The theory is supported by the observation that Kaposi's has its highest incidence in Zaire, the suspected country of origin of the current AIDS epidemic. However, subsequent discoveries have not supported this particular idea, as Dr Anne Bayley, a British surgeon in Zambia, has explained. She was puzzled by the first stories of Kaposi's appearance in the US. These cases were said to be untreatable — which made them quite unlike those of Dr Bayley's experience at the University Teaching Hospital in Lusaka. There she had found that most Kaposi's patients could be successfully treated with drugs. But the situation changed dramatically in 1983 when a new, aggressive form of the sarcoma suddenly appeared among her patients. None responded to treatment and all subsequently died. 'It was like coming home from work and finding that your spaniel had turned into a wolf. It was so against one's expectations,' she recalled in an interview in the *International Herald Tribune*.

Before then, nearly all Dr Bayley's Kaposi's sarcoma patients had been successfully treated by anti-cancer drugs, such as actinomycin D and vincristine. Afterwards, nearly all her new Kaposi's cases died within six months. These victims also showed unusual symptoms. They suffered severe weight loss, had difficulties with their breathing, and had particularly severe lesions on their skin. By 1984, Dr Bayley had 37 new Kaposi's patients, 22 of whom had the aggressive form.

But the crucial observation came when the new Kaposi's sufferers were tested for the AIDS virus. Nearly all were found to be HTLV3/LAV positive. It is a intriguing discovery. AIDS' association with a very special, new form of Kaposi's adds another crucial piece of evidence to the AIDS mystery, offering scientists a tantalizing new route for investigation. Indeed, the African AIDS epidemic may be particularly important in the fight against the disease. If its source can be located, then scientists may be able to learn how to deal with the virus.

At present, most scientists agree that Africa is indeed the source of the AIDS virus. They paint a fairly standard picture of the diseases's spread. For an unknown (but presumably lengthy) period of time there was an AIDS epidemic in Zaire, which eventually began to infect large numbers of people, perhaps around the mid-1970s. At that time, Zaire had close political links with Haiti and had been involved in large exchanges of personnel, particularly among military staff. Either through Zaireans visiting Haiti, or vice versa, the disease then spread to Haiti. Alternatively, some people suggest that Americans may have picked up the virus in Africa and spread it to Haiti.

After that, AIDS began to infect homosexuals, who have used Haiti as a favourite holiday resort for many years. (Some Haitians are believed to use male prostitution as a way of earning dollars from rich US visitors.) Once in America, the disease then spread into the other risk groups through contaminated blood. Shortly afterwards, Europe was hit by a double wave of infections. One came from the US and the other directly from Africa — for instance from

Zaire which, as the former Belgian Congo, has strong cultural and social links with Belgium.

This interpretation begs many questions. It has also caused a great deal of controversy. For one thing, it does not explain the reasons for the virus's recent emergence. If the disease was so well established in Zaire, why did it not spread to other countries before the 1970s? Scientists do not know the answer and point out that they have only very recently learned about the disease. However, most suspect that social factors were responsible for dislodging the disease, perhaps from a remote tribe in whom AIDS was either a recognized illness, or produced so many different symptoms that it was not recognized as an ailment in its own right. It could be the case that the carriers had — and may still have — some resistance to infection from the virus. This last possibility particularly intrigues scientists and entices many to make much closer and more detailed looks at AIDS in Africa.

Certainly early evidence did support the idea that AIDS had existed in Africa for a long time. By investigating blood samples taken in the past for other purposes and which were frozen because of their potential as a valuable new source of data, scientists found signs that the AIDS virus may have been infecting people since the early 1960s. Dr Harold Meyer of the US Food and Drug Administration studied blood taken from 144 children in the Upper Volta in 1963. His team reported finding signs of the AIDS virus — or something very like it — in the blood of two of these children. Other tests in Zaire, Uganda, and Kenya also produced evidence that an AIDS-like virus was infecting people's blood in the early 1970s.

These findings supported the idea that AIDS was established in Africa long before it struck in the US and Europe. But others have since questioned these results. Dr Richard Tedder of the Middlesex Hospital, London, believes that blood infected by malarial parasites and other infectious agents — a common problem in tropical countries — have produced many false positive readings in AIDS tests. Tropical blood is said to become 'sticky' and the problem gets worse the older the blood sample, so increasing the number of false positives in tests. 'I think many of the studies of early blood samples have produced a large number of false positive readings', says Dr Tedder. 'I think they should be re-examined now. Personally, I believe AIDS is a new epidemic in Africa'.

Dr Tedder's views are shared by an increasing number of scientists, such as Dr G. Hunsmann who, together with a group of West German and Zambian doctors, carried out AIDS tests on more than 4,000 Africans in seven countries. Writing in a British medical journal, they reported: 'It would seem that the epidemic of AIDS in Africa started at about the same time as, or even later than, the epidemics in America and Europe. Our results do not support the hypothesis that AIDS originated in Africa.'

These disagreements are seized upon by Africans anxious for evidence which suggests that AIDS does not come from Africa. 'There is no reason why we should take the blame for being the source of AIDS', says Dr Williams. 'In fact, there is just as much evidence to suggest that American tourists have been spreading it round the world. Just look at the figures. It's a city illness. That would fit the tourist hypothesis.' However, Dr Williams admitted that AIDS 'may have existed in an undisturbed state, or in a quiescent form in Africa. However, it took some other, external factor to dislodge it and send it across Africa and the rest of the world. That factor could be American tourists.'

In fact, scientists are divided about interpretations of AIDS' progress through Africa. Some believe it is an old disease and point out that it cannot have spread so widely in Africa in only four years. But what factor turned it into a worldwide epidemic? At present, they do not know. The other camp maintains that the AIDS epidemic is as new in Africa as it is the West. If so, then the virus must have mutated from an old, previously safe form. But how did that happen? Again scientists cannot say, though they do acknowledge the answer could be crucial in preventing similar epidemics in future.

The clues about the virus's origins are sketchy. Nevertheless, researchers are sure they provide important pointers to HTLV3/LAV's origins. For instance, Dr Max Essex of the Harvard School of Public Health, S. M'Boup of Dakar University in Senegal and Francis Barin of the Hôpital Bretonneau in Tours, France, have reported in the journal *Science* that they have found a retrovirus in wild African green monkeys that is very similar to the AIDS virus. The scientists believe that the virus may somehow have crossed from monkeys to men and women.

Support for this theory was found by Essex and his colleagues when they tested blood from prostitutes in Senegal. They found some had been infected by the monkey virus and not by the closely related AIDS virus. Yet none of this virus-positive group showed any symptoms of AIDS or AIDS-related conditions. Neither do green monkeys, who seem to be able to carry the virus quite happily. The scientists suggest that the monkey virus may be non-toxic but may have mutated in humans to acquire its deadly, destructive attributes. How the virus passed from monkeys to humans is more difficult to explain. However, green monkeys are a common pest in many parts of Africa and perhaps by biting or scratching a human they could have passed on the virus. In support of his theory, Essex also reported at the 'AIDS in Africa' conference that he had found that the African HTLV3/LAV strain is slightly different from the strain which affects victims in the US. He also found that African HTLV3/LAV behaves more like the monkey virus in laboratory experiments.

The work of Essex, M'Boup and Barin did not find favour with the African delegation at the conference, however. 'Why do they not look for a monkey in the US?', asked Dr David Benoni of Gabon. 'AIDS started there and could well have been brought to Africa by Americans.' He was backed by the rest of the African delegation. At a separate meeting there, they signed a statement which said that the symposium papers 'did not show any conclusive evidence that AIDS originated in Africa. It is a global problem and not an Africa problem alone', they argued. 'Therefore efforts directed to finding an African association with AIDS do not contribute to future control programmes.'

Their argument makes sense. AIDS is indeed a worldwide problem. However, its prevalence in Africa offers unique insights into the virus's behaviour — in particular the apparent ease with which it spreads between men and women. (Significantly, the African delegates especially acknowledged in their statement that 'heterosexual promiscuity is one of the high risk factors for AIDS'.) It is crucial that scientists be freely allowed to study AIDS in Africa and to pursue every aspect of its spread there, even if it means upsetting African sensitivities. Both the West and Africa have too much to lose.

If AIDS can spread as easily among heterosexuals in the rest of the world as it can among Africans, then the US and Europe may be on the brink of a dangerous new threat to public health. And even if AIDS is not quite such a serious threat in the West, Africa can still learn a great deal from the expertise of US and European scientists.

7

The Risks

Arthur is prepared for death. An AIDS victim who was diagnosed as a sufferer in 1985 and who featured so disturbingly in the sensational coverage of the Wormwood Scrubs AIDS scare stories, he is aware of the remorseless nature of his condition.

'Statistically, I know I am going to die, though medically I feel fit,' he says. 'It is still difficult to accept that my time is limited and I can never suppress the hope that something might save me at the last minute. Nevertheless, within myself, I know I am going to die.' Coming to terms with the fact has not been easy for Arthur. 'I have tried to talk about my death with my children and with my close friends. They won't listen. They say I am being morbid. But I am not. I am being realistic. I am going to die and, not surprisingly, I think about that a lot of the time. I am trying to come to terms with death but people won't let me.'

Arthur's problem is sad and distressing, although, in comparison with other AIDS victims, he has adjusted well. Among others, the diagnosis of AIDS has had catastropic effects. Some sufferers have attempted suicide, sometimes successfully. Their problems, and those of Arthur, are one of the least publicized aspects of the AIDS story. They reveal the intense psychological pressures that affect people facing a virtual sentence of death; who must also deal with a largely uncaring society; and who often feel intense guilt because they may have passed on the virus to lovers and friends.

For those diagnosed as carriers, but in whom no symptoms have developed, the pressures are not so severe or immediate, but they are still considerable. Their problems are summed up by Dr Donald Acheson, Britain's chief medical officer:

> The personal and social implications of HTLV-3 infection for the infected person are calamitous. A male must accept the likelihood of being infective sexually for an indefinite period, possibly for life, in addition to suffering from a potentially fatal condition for which there is no effective treatment and for which there is an uncertain but extended latent period.
>
> All infected persons face the risk of stigma and of being ostracized — like children in the USA who are refused entrance to school and adults who may lose jobs, or be refused employment, without justification.

Trying to alleviate victimization and suffering should be a priority for any caring society. But counselling AIDS sufferers has another important function — to help prevent others from becoming infected. On their own, victims cannot be expected to remain celibate, and to take all the pressure of ensuring the containment of the AIDS virus. They need support and help. Lonely and rejected people may easily take comfort in sex or in new relationships which might cause then the virus to spread.

The problem is revealed again through the story of Arthur. 'For nine months after finding out I had AIDS, I completely lost my sex drive. I just wasn't interested in it any more. Then one evening, an old lover phoned and suggested we have "safe sex".'

Many support groups for gays and virus carriers, such as the Terrence Higgins Trust, now urge homosexuals to practice 'safe sex' as a way of ensuring that HTLV3/LAV is not passed on to others. These methods exclude any activities that might cause the exchange of body fluids, in particular the emission of semen into the anus which is considered to carry a specially high risk of transmitting the AIDS virus. As substitutes, they recommend acts such as dry kissing (i.e., not involving the exchange of saliva) mutual masturbation, and body rubbing. 'I had never been turned on by things like that. However, I did agree to meet him and try safe sex', says Arthur. 'It was a disaster. In fact, it was horrible. I kept remembering what sort of sex we used to have. But now he knew I had AIDS — for I had made a point of telling all my past lovers when I was first diagnosed. Every time I went to touch him, he instinctively shrank back a little. Unconsciously, he felt I was contagious. He couldn't hide it. It was awful.'

Despite the misery of that experience, it did arouse sexual feelings that Arthur had suppressed for so long:

Shortly afterwards, I was going to work in the morning and was standing on the platform of my local station when I met this man's eyes. Our gazes held for just a little longer than normal. We started talking and arranged to meet later.

It was extremely pleasant, and in a way quite like old times. But at the back of my mind, I was thinking: 'What can I do? I can't tell this guy that I have got suspected AIDS, it will completely freak him.' In the end, I just could not bring myself to tell him.

Since that encounter, Arthur and his new friend have met regularly but have only practised safe sex:

It is much better now. He still doesn't know I have AIDS and doesn't pull away when I touch him. I know I have been a bit devious but really it was necessary. I couldn't face the thought of him shrinking back from me as well. Of course, I must tell him I have got AIDS. But again I will be a bit devious. I will suggest that we both take the test, 'to be on the safe side', and then I will act in a very surprised way when it shows I am carrying the virus antibodies. It is the only solution that I can see. I must do something, that is certain. The problem will just get worse and worse, the more I see of him.

Arthur's dilemma underlines one of the major risks in the battle to prevent the spread of the AIDS virus. Apparently infected and infectious for life, carriers like Arthur are being required by society to shoulder a massive burden to take responsibility for containing the virus.

'If you live a gay life — with drugs, late nights, parties and sex — it is very hard when you are suddenly expected to give all that up. People need help in getting over the isolation', says Jonathan Grimshaw, of Body Positive. 'Gays often begin to feel like social lepers even with other homosexuals. Gay men use casual sexual contacts as the starting points for new friendships and emotional attachments. When they find they are carrying the virus, this is no longer easy. To ask for "safe sex" is difficult and invites rejection.'

The possibility of rejection from people who should provide most comfort can put enormous strain on a virus carrier. 'He may rebel against an impossible situation, reject the source of his anxiety, and attempt to escape from his dilemma through extremes of behaviour — in particular increased sexual activity — with all the risks that that entails', warns Grimshaw.

But homosexual AIDS virus carriers are not the only ones being put under such pressure. In fact, every AIDS carrier is put in a similar position, though some have better support and are not treated as 'social lepers'. All are being required by society to completely change their lives, however. And the risks they pose are a major worry for doctors.

Pregnant women make up one such group. A Royal College of Obstetricians and Gynaecologists report warns that any woman carrying the AIDS virus should now be 'strongly advised' not to have a baby. They also recommend that women found to be AIDS virus carriers, and who are already pregnant should be offered abortions, while women from high risk groups, such as drug takers, should be screened for HTLV3/LAV as soon as they are found to be pregnant.

The report by Dr Pinching and Dr Donald Jeffries, also of St Mary's Hospital, London, highlights two main reasons for these drastic recommendations. First, it has been found there is a high risk that a child born to an AIDS-positive mother will be infected by the virus. Of these babies, about half will develop AIDS within two years. In addition, babies of infected mothers are also more likely to be congenitally malformed. There is also a danger to the mother's health while carrying a child, say Dr Pinching and Dr Jeffries. It is believed that pregnancy actually increases the chances of her developing AIDS or a related condition.

Once again, pressures are being brought to bear on particular sections of society in attempts to limit AIDS cases. In cases involving pregnant women, such measures have obvious direct benefits for the mothers themselves, and are likely to be accepted. That may not be the case with other groups, however, One extremely worrying example is provided by drug users. They lack even the support that exists for homosexuals. Nor is the evidence strong that they would take notice of advice or support if it were offered to them.

As one drug addict, appearing on the Thames Television *TV Eye* programme 'AIDS and You', said about heroin users: 'They really don't care. If they aren't able to get any sort of help, their reaction is likely to be "I don't care. I will just go out and spread it anyway".' Similar problems and attitudes may occur with prostitutes who become infected. Yet the reactions of these groups to infection is crucial. With no cures or vaccines in sight only acceptance of voluntary measures, or the imposition of draconian restraints on 'risky' activities, are likely to halt the spread of AIDS. And these measures will only work with people who are aware of their infectivity. 'The trouble is that because of the long latency period of AIDS, some people just don't know they are infected', adds Dr James Curran, of the CDC.

The risks represented by uncertain reactions to appeals for responsibility form only one crucial variable that will determine the course of the AIDS epidemic. Other factors include the dangers to blood transfusion services. As Professor Jeffrey Laurence states: 'Because a small fraction of AIDS carriers do not produce detectable amounts of antibody to the virus, current procedures for screening blood donors may not entirely eliminate the risk of infection from blood transfusions'. Such risks are probably minor ones, however. A more important factor is the degree to which the virus can pass between men and women.

This critical problem is summed up well by Dr Acheson,

the man in charge of controlling Britain's response to the AIDS crisis. A careful, and well-respected Belfast-born epidemiologist, he was appointed to the post of chief medical officer at the Department of Health in 1983, just as the first signs of the spread of AIDS spread within the UK were emerging. His cautious assessment of the risks posed by the virus's spread reflects both his nature as a scientist and as a senior civil servant. His analysis is also extremely interesting:

> The key issue which will determine the eventual scale of the AIDS epidemic, and which highlights the importance of health education, is the ease of transmission of infection as a result of heterosexual intercourse. A small number of female partners of bisexual males and of haemophiliacs have become infected — which suggests that transmission of infection from male to female, presumably by semen in the course of vaginal intercourse, can take place.
>
> As far as transmission from female to male, the evidence is conflicting. In New York City, in spite of a large number of AIDS cases in female prostitutes who have contracted the disease through drug abuse, there have been only 28 cases out of a total of 3,354 cases among men who did not admit to either homosexual intercourse or drug abuse or belonging to another high risk group.

Other studies have suggested that female to male transmission occurs, but Dr Acheson believes other factors, such as drug abuse, have not been satisfactorily ruled out. Nevertheless, he adds — significantly — that 'although American data suggests homosexual intercourse is the most important means of the sexual spread of HTLV-3 infection, it would be wrong to assume that heterosexual intercourse will not in the long run take on a significant role — and it is important that everyone should fully appreciate this point'.

Other scientists are more sure of AIDS' future heterosexual spread. For them, the evidence from Africa, and from a few cases in America and Europe, is highly revealing. 'I think it would be utterly foolish to think that

AIDS is going to be confined to gays in the West and to people of both sexes in Africa', says Professor Robin Weiss. 'It's going to spread to both sexes in the West too.'

Hard evidence to support this assertion is scarce. However, Professor Weiss's views are backed by an increasing number of other scientists. 'I have seen so many cases of men who have contracted AIDS and who insist they could only have got it from prostitutes', says Dr Dalgleish.

'I can see no reason why these men should lie. They have developed an extremely serious condition. There is nothing to be gained in denying homosexual relations they might have had. Yet they insist they have had none. I think the inference is clear — this is a straightforward sexually transmitted disease.

One study that provides support was carried out by the US Army. Its doctors investigated a group of soldiers who were found to carry the AIDS virus. On questioning, only 17 per cent of these soldiers admitted to homosexuality, while 37 per cent admitted they had had sex with prostitutes. However, scientists — including Dr Acheson — say the possibility of drug abuse, or even of homosexuality, still have not been properly ruled out in this particular study.

Other researchers are beginning to find new clues. At the AIDS in Africa conference, when a general question was raised about evidence of a Western heterosexual spread which might parallel Africa's, several US doctors spoke of intriguing preliminary studies of cases of men becoming infected after sleeping with the former female partners of virus positive haemophiliacs and drug addicts. These studies are in their infancy and certainly do not constitute an overwhelming case for those who believe that a widespread heterosexual spread of AIDS is imminent. But as these adherents point out, the virus simply has not had enough time to get into the heterosexual population and spread.

Nevertheless, support has come from a particularly intriguing analysis carried out by Professor Julian Peto — an epidemiologist, like Dr Acheson. His conclusions differ very greatly from his counterpart's. 'I look at the case for the heterosexual spread of AIDS from the opposite point of view', he says. 'As far as I can see there isn't any evidence that it is *not* going to spread heterosexually, while there is a lot of strong evidence that it *is* going to do so. Just look at what is going on in Africa. There are absolutely no grounds for ignoring its heterosexual spread there and for believing that it won't happen here.'

Those seeking evidence that AIDS will spread among the general population have always been confounded by the fact that the percentage of Western heterosexual victims, among total numbers of AIDS cases, has remained constant — at about one or two per cent since the epidemic began. Shouldn't that figure have risen by now if AIDS is going to affect men and women alike, ask the optimists?

Seeking comfort in this observation will do no good, says Professor Peto. Taking the same set of figures for New York AIDS victims that was quoted by Dr Acheson, he comes to a very different conclusion in his analysis. He points out that other categories of AIDS victims also cover people infected through heterosexual activity. For instance, the group identified simply as 'no known risks' must surely be made up of heterosexuals. Similarly, those known to come from African countries must also be counted as heterosexually infected victims. 'When you add up these figures you actually find that about 200 of New York's AIDS victims are heterosexuals', says Peto.

'Now that still might not seem to be a lot out of a total of more than 3,000 AIDS victims in the city, until you think how many AIDS victims there are in Britain — about 200. That means New York alone has got as big a heterosexual AIDS epidemic as Britain has in total. So to say the disease is not beginning to manifest itself among heterosexuals to any extent would be quite incorrect.' But Professor Peto does not end his disturbing analysis there. He also points out that since the beginning of the AIDS epidemic in the US, cases have consistently increased at a fixed rate, with numbers doubling every six to eight months. This means that numbers are increasing roughly threefold every year; tenfold every two years; and therefore by one hundredfold every four years. This is an approximate calculation. However, it does reflect the true picture. In the US in 1980, there were 46 cases of AIDS. By 1984, there were 4,293. 'That leaves you with a piece of simple arithmetic', says Peto. 'If the level of heterosexual AIDS cases in America is about one per cent of the total — a conservative estimate — that means in four years you are going to have the same number of heterosexual AIDS cases as the current total American figure. At present, that figure is more than 15,000 — a very frightening level'.

Professor Peto acknowledges that his calculation is 'a very speculative prediction'. But he adds: 'There is nothing to show that it is not true. All the evidence is consistent with its accuracy. AIDS spread just that way among heterosexuals in Africa, after all.' He adds that the evidence can already be seen that a heterosexual epidemic as large as the present homosexual one will occur by the end of the decade. 'For instance, you would expect that early signs of infection would occur among promiscuous heterosexuals — and that is what we are beginning to see.'

One important factor that will have delayed the onset of the disease among heterosexuals is the make-up of the original risk groups. By accident, they are mostly men — male homosexuals; haemophiliacs, who are almost always male; and drug takers, who are predominantly male. That has distorted statistics in a particularly interesting way. If most of the first AIDS victims and virus carriers are male then there can be few female victims and carriers who can then infect men heterosexually. Because there are a lot more males with the virus, there will be a lot more women picking up the virus from them compared with the number of women who can give the virus to men. And this is exactly what you find. Of the 52 heterosexually infected AIDS victims in New York, fifty were women, and two were men. This difference occurs because there were few infected women to give the virus to men. Scientists like Professor Peto believe this situation will not last for much longer.

Really, what evidence is there that AIDS is not spread heterosexually? I can find very little. Indeed, the only unanswered question is how quickly it will spread into the general population. That will depend on future levels of promiscuity and the rate of female to male transmission. I don't think the spread will occur as quickly as the one that occurred among Western heterosexuals or among African men and women. Nevertheless it will happen.

Certainly, the disease's passage through present risk populations has been astonishing. In five years the virus has spread to 72 countries and infected millions. 'We never thought AIDS was going to spread this rapidly because this sort of virus is difficult to transmit', says Gallo. 'Nevertheless, inexorably, it has affected country after country.' Whether a similar rapid spread through Western heterosexuals is about to occur cannot yet be answered, although Professor Peto's analysis is alarming.

'At the moment, AIDS is not a problem among heterosexuals to any great degree in Europe' says Dr John Harris. 'However, that is no reason for being complacent. It would be prudent to expect such a spread and be prepared for it. My advice to men and women now would be to limit numbers of sexual partners.'

To some that is a rudimentary precaution , to others it is an alarmist notion. Either way, it is clear that some careful thinking must now be done about measures to contain the spread of AIDS.

8

The Answers

Zelda Rubinstein is only 4 ft 3 in (1.3 metres) tall but she is a big name in Los Angeles. Her diminutive features are displayed on television, on billboards, on leaflets, and in newspapers throughout the city. Zelda is an actress and had a lead role in the film *Poltergeist*. But her fame has since been made outside Hollywood. It rests on her portrayal of 'Mother', the central character in a state-funded health education campaign aimed at reducing AIDS' spread in Los Angeles.

'Mother' delivers television homilies, backed up by newspaper stories, adverts and leaflets, to her wayward 'children', the homosexuals of the West Coast. Dressed in frilly apron and bedroom slippers, the tiny figure of 'Mother' waves a wooden spoon as she imparts her messages: 'Don't forget your rubbers (condoms)', and 'Don't let a hot number get you to do unsafe things in bed'.

The presentation is lighthearted, but the aim is deadly serious. It is to persuade the one million gays who live in Los Angeles to adopt 'safe sex' practices that will cut down the transmission of the AIDS virus. So far 'Mother' has received an enthusiastic response. Indeed, she has become a cult figure and is constantly invited to appear in gay bars and discos to deliver her message. Signs are emerging that gays have been listening and reacting to her warnings — and to similar ones from many other anti-AIDS campaigns in California. There are no precise surveys of Los Angeles gays, but in neighbouring San Francisco, about 80 per cent of homosexuals have reported they are limiting numbers of partners and are avoiding risky practices such as anal intercourse.

It is one of the most encouraging developments in the

battle against AIDS and is certainly desperately needed. Every day, in Los Angeles and San Francisco, four new cases of AIDS are diagnosed and two people die of the disease. Figures like that, repeated throughout the world, would represent a dreadful level of suffering in years to come. Limiting the virus's spread to other gays is therefore an obvious first step in the war against AIDS. But will this new austerity among gays make a difference? Tony Whitehead is not so sure. 'Gays in San Francisco have responded well and have cut down on multiple partnering', he says. 'But it is too late. If you look at infections in the city, you find that at least 50 per cent, probably 75 per cent of them, are now carrying the virus. That means only a quarter are not virus positive.'

Apart from the dreadful consequences for individuals, such a massive pool of infected gays makes the disease's containment very difficult. In the past, when there were only a few carriers in the city, San Franciscan gays needed many partners to run a serious risk of catching the AIDS virus. Now, with three quarters of the city's gays as carriers, a single encounter produces a high chance of infection. This problem will spread to other cities and countries, says Professor Peto.

AIDS has such a long latency period, and has so many symptomless carriers, that people do not appreciate the danger and take drastic action until it is too late. Look at Britain. Most AIDS cases and virus carriers live in London. Gays elsewhere in the UK do not think they are at risk — and probably will not be until the virus is established in their part of the country. By then it will be too late. So it is not enough for London gays to adopt drastic, 'safe sex' measures. That action must be taken by gays elsewhere, *before* the virus spreads to them. However, I doubt if they will because they don't think they are at risk. Indeed, it is silly to expect them to change their lifestyles just because it has been announced it is a good idea.

Only drastic action can halt AIDS' spread, says Peto. 'Otherwise we will be left with a massive permanent problem. Of course, drastic measures may not work, but then again they might. If nothing else, people will at least understand the seriousness of the problem.' The drastic measures favoured by Professor Peto include the introduction of a 'green card' system for gays. Possession would show a person was free of the AIDS virus and was safe as a sex partner. 'It's very sensible. Gays must be tested or at least should be urged to do so. The green card system would put just the right kind of pressure on them.'

Professor Peto stresses that his scheme would only work with co-operation from the gay community. But the pressure should be strong. Gentle encouragement is not enough, he says. 'Do gay leaders really think that merely asking people to give up risky sex is enough? If they do, it is quite unrealistic.'

But gay activists find the idea quite unacceptable. 'There isn't much difference between tattooing carriers and compelling other gays to carry "virus-free" cards showing they are not risks in my view', says Tony Whitehead. The disagreement reveals one of the major problems that have arisen over attempts to combat AIDS — protecting the civil liberties of minority groups while ensuring that disease control measures are effective.

In fact, many gay community leaders, and others involved in counselling victims, advise against taking the AIDS antibody test in the first place. 'Just waiting for the results is bad enough,' says Les Lattner, of the Terrence Higgins Trust. 'They can take weeks to arrive and that can be nerve-racking on its own.' Others point out the serious disadvantages of a virus positive diagnosis — possible loss of life insurance (and even mortgage if it is linked to a life insurance policy), accommodation and even jobs. As a result, many counsellors privately advise risk group members not to take the test. Their only exception is for those planning families and whose children might be affected.

'If you are in a high risk group, you should take

precautions anyway — such as curtailing numbers of sexual partners', says one professional counsellor. 'These precautions are the same whether you are a carrier or not. They cut the risks of you spreading or contracting AIDS. So what's the point of taking the test? You will gain nothing. You are only likely to lose your life insurance cover, job and accommodation. And don't forget, there is slight but definite rate of a false positive result with the test — so you may even be told you are carrier when you are not.'

Similar fears are expressed in America. Gay groups such as the Gay Men's Health Crisis distribute leaflets that warn that 'the test can be almost as devastating as the disease'. The leaflets state:

> The new test for antibodies to the AIDS virus doesn't tell you very much of anything. It only indicates that you have been exposed to the virus. What it can do is frightening.
>
> Imagine if your health insurance company found out that your test came back positive, they might cancel your policy. Even your job and home may be at risk. Names might be reported to the government and find their way onto a master list.

In Britain, worries are also expressed about confidentiality. Many support organizations warn that if potential carriers have decided that they must take the test, they should not use a general practitioner who may reveal results to an employer. (Many GPs privately admit they would give this information if asked by a company's medical officer.) The next development could then be loss of employment. Instead, the test should be taken at a sexual disease clinic where there is likely to be better confidentiality.

Many doctors object. 'We have got to know if a patient is virus positive', says one London GP. 'The knowledge is necessary to ensure proper medical treatment. For instance, we might give him live vaccines that could have serious effects on him.' (A live vaccine is made up of still living but weakened microbes which give immunity to a disease. In patients who are immune-depressed, this could produce side-effects.)

But gays are adamant that their civil liberties must not be eroded. And they point to the example of Enserch, the parent company of Dallas Lone Star Gas Company. It has started screening current and prospective workers in employee cafeterias. Anyone found to be virus positive will either be moved or not given a job. To force a person to take an AIDS test and then to refuse to give them employment after the devastating revelation of carrier status is brutal and inhuman, say gays.

Such arguments do not impress Professor Peto: 'Checking the spread of infection is not for the benefit of those already infected. It is for the benefit of society, which takes priority over gay rights and over the enormous unhappiness caused by telling people they are virus positive.' Professor Peto goes on to say: 'We must face this issue. These people may be the victims of an epidemic but we cannot afford to keep them ignorant and cheerful while the disease spreads. I think it is preferable to let them suffer.'

These sentiments are a little too strong for other scientists including Britain's Dr Acheson. 'I think it's essential to work with the gay community rather than against them', he said in an interview in *The Times*. 'If you react to the people at risk in a hostile way, they will be alienated and will not come forward for diagnosis and advice and may be tempted to behave in an irresponsible way.'

In fact, gays have generally behaved very responsibly. This is certainly the case in San Francisco, one of the cities worst affected by AIDS, where an estimated 10,000 young men will probably die of the disease. As Alex Brummer, *The Guardian*'s correspondent in California put it: 'As the years slip by, the risque, hedonistic orgies of the early 1980s have given way to the new puritanism and funerals of the late 1980s'.

In San Francisco, gay groups run counselling services, hold seminars, make television documentaries, and operate switchboard services to answer questions from a city population that still regards AIDS as a perplexing and terrifying phenomenon. One switchboard, run by the San Francisco AIDS Foundation, receives more than 5,000 calls a month.

'Chuck, a victim with scabbed lips whose blood no longer clots properly, runs the switchboard', states Brummer in a despatch from the city. 'Over a half-an-hour period, he fields a call from a woman with small scarlet, but harmless, bumps on her body; a lover whose gay partner has been diagnosed with an AIDS infection of the brain and who fears for his own mortality; a married man who wonders whether casual homosexual experiences have infected his wife; and a woman who is worried about allowing a gay friend to play with her children now that he has AIDS.'

However, the heart of the city's response to AIDS lies at the city's general hospital. There doctors have adopted a policy of keeping AIDS victims in the community for as long as possible. Only when the ravaging effects of Kaposi's sarcoma or wasting attacks of PCP pneumonia have reached a critical level are victims admitted and given a bed in the hospital's luxurious AIDS ward. Other sufferers attend the hospital's special outpatient clinic where every month doctors treat more than 1,000 doomed young men.

Despite the careful, compassionate treatment of San Francisco doctors, the worldwide picture is depressing. At present, little can be done except postpone inevitable death by treating any opportunistic infections while gays and authorities tussle over containment tactics. But what about less fatalistic approaches? Surely scientists can develop cures, treatments or vaccines? As Samual Broder, chairman of an AIDS drug evaluation committee at the US National Institutes of Health, says: 'It is important to start with a working assumption that AIDS is a curable disease. If a doctor believes that any given patient is incurable, that doctor will always be proved right'.

And researchers are indeed sure they will find cures and treatments. The important question is when? In the case of an AIDS vaccine, the answer is probably not for a very long time — perhaps not until the late 1990s. As for cures or treatments, it is extremely difficult to say when a really effective one will be developed. Much effort is being expended with occasional encouraging initial results. However, optimism has all too frequently been dashed. Promising treatments that have subsequently proved unsuccessful have included bone-marrow transplants and T-cell injections. Both were attempts to replenish depleted immune systems. However, the new cells were simply infected by the old ones, it appears. Patients have also been given interleukin-2 and interferons in bids to restore critical chemical messenger systems left crippled by infected T-helpers. Again, there was no success.

Other scientists have concentrated on drugs that counter reverse transcriptase — the chemical used by HTLV3/LAV to make DNA copies of itself. If this process could be blocked the virus could not make copies of itself and the virus spread would halt. Several drugs counteract reverse transcriptase, such as suramin, which is also used to treat tropical protozoal infections. Other drugs that can inhibit a virus's lifecycle include ribavirin, which has been used against cold and flu viruses; HPA-23; and alpha-interferon. Trials with all these drugs have been carried out on AIDS patients with little success so far. Scientists have found that the drugs can interfere with reverse transcriptase activity and viral replication. However, they also inhibit the growth of the body's own cells, particularly those of the immune system.

In the case of suramin, supressed levels of the AIDS virus were found in patients. However, there were also toxic side effects and as soon as treatments were stopped, the virus reappeared. Preliminary studies with HPA-23 produced similar results, despite French doctors' great hopes for the drug. Although HPA-23 appeared to suppress the virus, no clinical improvements could be observed in patients. However, more detailed tests are still being carried out.

The difficulties in using such drugs are summed up by Gallo: 'You want to kill reverse transcriptase — but you want to do it with specificity. You don't want to inhibit or interfere with normal proliferating cells. To my knowledge, nobody in the world has a good specific inhibitor of reverse transcriptase. We need more research and more help from the pharmaceutical industry.'

Such difficulties are understandable given the nature of the disease. The AIDS virus is extremely hard to erradicate because it actually becomes part of the cell it infects. The virus also infects the brain, and is therefore protected from many blood-borne drugs whose large molecules cannot pass through the blood-brain barrier. In addition, diagnosis of AIDS usually occurs after a patient's immune system has been depleted, so therapies must both destroy the virus and restore the immune system. Clearly, strategies involving combinations of drugs are needed, and doctors are already planning these. One scheme is to use drugs, such as isoprinosine and interleukin-2, which boost the immune system in conjunction with antiviral agents like suramin and ribavirin.

However, such trials have to be carefully planned. Researchers cannot simply test drugs in an indiscriminate manner just because AIDS is a terminal illness. If they did, it would be extremely difficult to spot the effects of a truly useful medicine among a welter of changing symptoms and case conditions. As Dr Anthony Fauci, director of the US National Institute of Allergy and Infectious Diseases, a centre for AIDS drug testing, said in a *Science* interview: 'If you start throwing drugs out in haphazard ways, the horrible thing that could happen is that in five years, we would still be running in circles. But if we do it in an orderly fashion, then we will still be able to eliminate something that definitely is not worthwhile and go on to the next thing.' Unproven drugs 'might start killing AIDS patients in their beds', he adds.

Caution mixed with urgency is clearly their best

approach, say scientists. After all, they are faced with an extraordinarily difficult task. An effective anti-AIDS drug must have no toxic side-effects, should be administered orally, and must be tolerated for long periods, perhaps for the rest of a patient's life. It is a tall order. Nevertheless, doctors have been encouraged by some developments — such as the discovery of azidothymidine. Developed by Burroughs Wellcome, it was first considered as a potential anti-AIDS drug when it was found to suppress the activity of a leukaemia retrovirus in mice.

Azidothymidine also works by inhibiting reverse transcriptase, but not in a direct manner. Starting from the observation that the AIDS virus's variable structure helped it to trick immune systems, scientists concluded that the reverse transcriptase was making mistakes in copying the virus. 'We decided that if the virus could fool us, then may be we could fool the virus', says one scientist involved with the project.

So they selected a drug that reverse transcriptase could use as one of its building blocks for making DNA copies of the virus — but with a crucial factor included. Azidothymidine is not a complete building block. It lacks crucial ingredients. As a result, when used by reverse transcriptase, incomplete copies of the virus are made. Trials in laboratories have been encouraging and scientists including Dr Broder, and Dani Bolognasi at Duke University in the US, have also reported encouraging responses from patients treated with azidothymidine. Scientists believe similar drugs will prove to be extremely important for treating AIDS patients in future. 'It is one of the most exciting developments there has been in the AIDS story,' acknowledges Gallo.

Such optimism suggests that eventually AIDS treatments will be developed, though speed of success remains an unknown quantity. But there is another approach — the creation of a vaccine that will immunize and protect virus-free individuals against future contact with HTLV3/LAV. In

1984, US Health and Human Services Secretary Margaret Heckler announced that such a vaccine would be ready within two years. It was a rash prediction, for scientists have since discovered so many hurdles in their path that they have postponed their likely vaccine delivery date until the end of the century.

Their caution is understandable. For one thing, the structure of the AIDS virus is highly variable which means that a vaccine's provision of immunity to one strain may prove to be useless against another. In addition, it appears the virus may be transmitted directly from cell to cell without having to reach the bloodstream. This behaviour may make it difficult for scientists to develop vaccines that could prepare the body to track down such a well-hidden virus.

On top of these woes, there are also difficulties in finding animals that react as humans do to the virus. Monkeys are the logical candidates and some do react to the AIDS virus, but in a highly variable, unpredictable way. The most stable, human-like response is found in the chimpanzee. However, the chimpanzee is a protected species and numbers are in short supply for medical research.

Even if a non-toxic version of the AIDS virus could be found, there could be problems if it was used as a vaccine when injected directly into humans because the cancer-causing nature of the retrovirus might still trigger tumours.

It sounds extremely gloomy. Nevertheless, researchers believe there may still be ways round these difficulties. The discovery that there are parts of the virus that do not change in different strains is encouraging as these parts might be used in a vaccine that would provide wide protection. The discovery, by Max Essex and colleagues, of the monkey virus similar to the AIDS virus has also raised hopes that a vaccine might be developed from it.

And then there is the example of Professor William Jarrett, of Glasgow University's veterinary pathology department. Professor Jarrett is the developer of a vaccine which successfully counters the effects of a retrovirus that causes the equivalent of AIDS in cats. Many scientists think his work offers great hope. Professor Jarrett first discovered that the retrovirus responsible for feline leukaemia also caused feline AIDS. At the time he made his discovery, retroviruses were thought to cause diseases, particularly cancers and leukaemias, in only a few animals, particularly birds. It was also thought that the virus passed only from parents to offspring.

'Then one day, we discovered a huge colony of cats which were kept by a woman in a house in Glasgow', recalls Professor Jarrett. 'We found that eight of them had feline leukaemia but none of them were related. The virus was clearly being passed on through normal contacts'. To their amazement, Professor Jarrett's team then found that most Glasgow cats showed signs that they had at one time been infected with the virus. Most survived, a few developed leukaemia, and some contracted an unusual immune disease — now known as feline AIDS — which blocked the cats' powers to fight diseases.

His work was some of the most important pioneering research which helped to prepare scientists for the onset of human AIDS in 1981. Indeed, by the time AIDS appeared, Professor Jarrett was already working on a vaccine to counter its feline equivalent (which cannot affect humans). Again the task was made extremely difficult by the behaviour of the retrovirus involved. The feline retrovirus appears to be able to somehow switch off natural defences which would normally spring into action to defend the cat from invading microbes.

After laborious research, Professor Jarret isolated a strain of the virus that did not behave in this way. It did not switch off the body's defences. This version was injected back into cats. Their immune systems were then triggered in preparation for later infections from the feline AIDS virus.

Professor Jarrett has now turned to the human AIDS

virus and he has begun collaborating on vaccine research with Gallo in Washington. Many British scientists believe it is a highly promising association. As one says: 'If those two cannot develop a human AIDS vaccine then God knows who can. They make a formidable team.' But at present, conventional medicine has little to offer those now affected. It is therefore not surprising that many AIDS victims have turned to alternative therapies for salvation — and sometimes with apparent success.

Two of the best publicized cases are Louie Nassaney and Tom Proctor from Los Angeles. Their battles against AIDS have been covered on both television and in the newspapers on both sides of the Atlantic. Disciples of 'metaphysical counsellor' Louise Hay, they maintain that their survival has been achieved through positive thinking'.

Nassaney became a body builder after being diagnosed as an AIDS victim — eventually winning a runner-up prize in a muscleman competition and its prize of a free holiday in the Bahamas. Proctor became a marathon runner to stay healthy and to raise funds for AIDS research. They have followed advice to 'love yourself, heal your body'. Treatments involve flute music, incantations, and a healing crystal which is held over the patient who then talks directly to his afflicted T-cells to persuade them to drive out the AIDS virus.

Nassaney, who initially suffered diarrhoea, fevers, drastic loss of weight and eyesight problems, eventually abandoned standard medical treatments for his symptoms. Instead, he 'prayed to the Lord' and began imagining that his Kaposi's sarcoma lesions were pencil marks that would slowly be rubbed out. Over the following six months the lesions slowly disappeared. Nassaney then turned to his depleted immune system, imagined his T-helper cells were white rabbits and dreamt they were multiplying. Shortly afterwards, he reported his weight was returning to its previous healthy levels.

Proctor similarly decided he would reject a 'curl-up-and-die' approach and took up marathon running instead. His efforts, made in conjunction with treatment from Louise Hay, subsequently won him a citation as an 'exemplary citizen' of West Hollywood for his fund-raising work.

Sceptics point out that in many diseases, including AIDS, there are cases of temporary remissions in which patients make 'miracle' recoveries, but who eventually succumb to their condition. In the absence of any other form of treatment, few doctors are publically willing to deride the two men's achievements, however.

Others fear that as AIDS spreads and more people fall ill, there may be thousands more victims who will turn to practioners who are thoroughly unscrupulous. Their suffering will only be made worse. Such problems underline the urgency of the hunt to find effective ways of combating AIDS.

9

The Future

Actor Rock Hudson is AIDS' most famous victim. His struggle for life and subsequent death in 1985 stunned America. For the first time, people who thought the disease a remote problem became aware of its remorseless effects. As a CDC official put it: 'What changed in America was that someone everyone knew became affected.' This new awareness did not stop prejudice, but it did galvanize the US Congress into providing generous research funds for scientists battling against the disease. Hudson's demise also added fuel to the AIDS panic. 'This disease is a greater threat to the human race than nuclear war', claimed one US politician, shortly after the actor's death.

Such silly exaggerations are unhelpful, for the human species is certainly capable of adapting and evolving to new diseases, no matter how savage their effects. Nevertheless, AIDS may yet cause widespread suffering and death. Defining the exact risks, in a calm rational way, has been difficult for both doctors and journalists. A sense of alarm, but not panic, is the proper, measured response — but this is hard to put across.

Just how widely will AIDS spread? Pessimists say it will affect heterosexuals in large numbers. They believe that by the early 1990s there may be 12,000 cases in Britain alone, with a further 500,000 people infected with the virus. Optimists say the disease's heterosexual spread will be limited and suggest figures will be only a tenth of those predicted by pessimists. Both sides put forward convincing arguments: optimists stressing 'caution', pessimists promoting 'realism'. And each can summon strong supporting evidence.

Optimists point out that there has been no variation in levels of heterosexual AIDS sufferers as a percentage of total numbers of victims since 1981. They also claim that the possibility of special factors affecting AIDS heterosexual spread in Africa has not yet been satisfactorily ruled out. It is also likely that female-to-male transmission of HTLV3/LAV is more difficult than male-to-male transmission. And it may even be possible that the AIDS virus strain in Africa is more virulent than the American strain.

For their part, the pessimists highlight a string of warning signs — for instance that a fifth of homosexuals in San Francisco have reported that they had sex with women between 1981 and 1985. With many of these men being virus positive, their female partners may already have formed a deadly bridging group.

The pessimists also point out that many prostitutes are now affected through drug abuse. For instance, in Miami, 40 per cent of a group of prostitutes were found to be AIDS virus positive — forming another dangerous bridging group. Similarly, studies of virus carriers in the US Army have revealed that there are more soldiers who report heterosexual promiscuity as a probable source of their infection than there are soldiers who blame homosexual promiscuity.

On more general issues, the optimists and pessimists are also clearly divided. The former argue that AIDS is not really very infectious and is probably harder to pass on than a disease like hepatitis B, which also affects people with many different sex partners and which infects the blood of many drug takers. Indeed, around 5 per cent of those infected with the hepatitis B may die of their condition but no-one threatens to close schools, sack carriers, or tattoo victims because of their condition. The panic over AIDS has grossly exaggerated its dangers, say the optimists.

But the pessimists answer back by pointing out that AIDS has many other deadly attributes. The virus's capacity to lie undetected in the body for months or years means victims can pass it on in ignorance. In addition, the virus's apparent capacity for indefinite survival in the blood means a permanent pool of asymptomatic carriers is being created — a very dangerous development for any disease.

On balance, it is clear that AIDS must now be treated as a cause for very serious concern. As Jeremy Lawrence editor of *New Society* states: 'This is the biggest public health hazard we currently face — far worse than more fashionable concerns like lead in petrol or additives in food'.

The main fears now centre on the discovery that the AIDS virus attacks the central nervous system, producing speech disorders, personality changes, coma and death. Many scientists say these effects may greatly increase death rates from their present minimum estimate of 10 per cent of virus carriers. Some say privately that it could rise to between 50 and 90 per cent. Others merely state that the general outlook for carriers is poor. For instance, Dr Tedder says 'the future for virus positive people may be pretty bleak'.

The impact of the disease therefore looks grim — both in personal and financial terms. Already, AIDS is having a staggering effect on America's health services bill. By the end of 1985, cases were being reported at the average rate of ten a day at the CDC in Atlanta.

This means that by 1990, the disease could be costing America several billion dollars a year. Figures prepared by the CDC and the San Francisco Department of Public Health show that hospital bills for the 10,000 American AIDS victims diagnosed by May 1985 will eventually total $1.4 billion. This comes close to America's spending on lung cancer treatments — $1.6 billion. In fact, AIDS now kills as many young men in America as their other top causes of death, heart disease and cancer. It is also responsible for more deaths than crashes or suicides among young men. Such is the level of suffering that Nobel Peace Prize Winner

Mother Teresa says she wants to open an AIDS hospice in New York for victims that include affected prisoners.

And with the AIDS epidemic in Europe lagging behind the US by about three or four years, it is expected that similar stories and figures will be repeated there before the end of the decade. The statistics are dispiriting. But behind them lie the personal tragedies. All AIDS victims' stories are sad and distressing. Some have been anguishing. One particularly revealing story concerns John who died of AIDS on Christmas Day 1985. Tim McGirk described his last days in *The Sunday Times*.

John was infected during factor VIII treatments for haemophilia and subsequently was affected by PCP. For three years his treatments included 'surgical implants, chemotherapy, drugs with poisonous side-effects and over 400 blood tests', says McGirk. Eventually John vowed never to return to hospital. Before he died, John suffered deep depression. Bedridden and growing weaker, he became convinced — wrongly — that his wife Meg was being unfaithful. He showed signs of brain infection and also became incontinent. Eventually John, a former Princeton University oarsman, died, aged thirty, his weight having plunged from 195lb to 135lb (88Kg to 61Kg).

There are some particularly revealing aspects to John's death. For one thing, although advised not to have intercourse with his wife to prevent the transmission of AIDS, it was discovered that they had had sex after infection but before diagnosis of his condition. However, he did not pass on the virus. Meg has been tested several times and has been found to be virus free. 'I am living proof that AIDS is a difficult disease to catch', she told McGirk.

Secondly, Meg found, to her surprise, that she had no difficulty finding an undertaker for her husband's corpse. 'The disease has claimed so many males on America's eastern coast that body-handlers have become blasé', says McGirk.

Thirdly, and most importantly, there were the

psychological and neurological aspects of John's condition. As with other patients, these are quite separate. The first is a reaction to the onset of a wasting fatal illness. The second is caused directly by HTLV3/LAV attacking the brain. Discriminating between them is very difficult, for the symptoms are often very similar. Understanding them is of critical importance, however, for knowledge of the former may help to alleviate the immediate suffering of victims, while information on the latter may reveal how the virus is attacking in the brain and may help in the development of new treatments.

A graphic description of the psychological aspects of AIDS is given by Christopher Spence. Discussing the death of a friend from the disease, Spence says it was like watching a man fight with his hands tied behind his back. His friend, Frank, suffered guilt as a working-class man who was gay. Spence believes this made him vulnerable when trying to combat the disease. 'A chronic feeling that you would like to die on the one hand, and that you deserve to die on the other, is hardly the best basis for resisting infection, for dealing with the terror of a life-threatening disease, and for coping with the fact that almost everyone around you — family, friends, doctors, nurses, and fellow patients — is terrified too.'

In fact, AIDS has unique psychological characteristics, say Wolcott, Fawzy and Pasnau. Diagnosis can induce anxiety, depression, social withdrawal because of stigmatization, apathy, pathological denial of diagnosis that leads to desperate attempts for other medical opinion, suicides, and 'excessive risk-taking behaviour, including drug abuse and participation in physically dangerous activities in apparent attempts to master the anxiety and sense of vulnerability precipitated by diagnosis'. Those associated with the patient also suffer. Families feel grief and 'cumulative physical and emotional exhaustion' in caring for the victim. Parents of gay victims suffer guilt because they feel their sons' conditions somehow reflect failures in their parenting. Similarly, patients' lovers go through intense guilt and stress.

The other behavioural changes — those caused by the virus's attacks on brain tissue — include dementia, delirium, language disorders, lethargy, cerebral haemorrhages, blindness, and coma. It is a disturbing list to add to an already lengthy catalogue of ailments. As Professor Peto puts it: 'If you wanted to design a bug for a horror science fiction film, you couldn't really top the AIDS virus'.

Small wonder then that some people have interpreted the onset of AIDS as an act of biblical retribution visited upon gays for their hedonistic, sinful ways. Today the evidence of AIDS' heterosexual impact is far too strong to support that notion. But the disease has certainly produced a profound impact on homosexual society. As Richard Fisher, author of the advice book, *AIDS: Your questions answered*, says of homosexual men, they are 'a recently liberated subculture that has danced a kind of charmed ballet for the better part of two decades. Now the sarabande has suddenly become a *danse macabre.'*

Only time will tell if that same *danse macabre* will be danced by the rest of the world. Measures can be taken to diminish risks but hopes must be tempered with realism. Past pleas for celibacy, to reduce spreads of other sexually transmitted diseases, have usually been ignored. And although AIDS has such a terrible reputation surpassing even cancer as a doctor's most feared diagnosis, there is still a dangerous tendency for people to view it as 'someone else's problem', as Dr Pinching points out. They may not find comfort in such thoughts for much longer.

Index